ACHIEVEMENTS IN MEDICINE

ACHIEVEMENTS IN MEDICINE

Achievements in Medicine
1974–1989

In honour of
Professor David Todd

Department of Medicine
University of Hong Kong

Rayson Huang Lecture Theatre, University of Hong Kong
25 November 1989

Published for

Department of Medicine, University of Hong Kong

by

Hong Kong University Press

ISBN 962-209-248-9

Printed in Hong Kong by Liang Yu Printing Factory Ltd.

CONTENTS

達者爲師今古同
安能煮酒定英雄
輝煌此日庭中果
教誨當年耳畔鐘
授我藝深征頑疾
任他池淺養蛟龍
滿逾廿載酬何價
送別依依兩袖風

己巳年陳文岩題
於香江

Poem by Dr. M.K. Chan, composed for the occasion.

ACKNOWLEDGEMENTS

We would like to thank all who contributed reviews on achievements in each subspecialty and produced their manuscripts with very short notice. The invaluable assistance of the following secretaries are much appreciated: Vicky Lee, Jenny Watt, Susie Yim, Theresa Tong, Monica Chan, Shirla Tam, Karis Larm and Angela Poon.

The professional advice and efficiency of production of this commemorative volume by Mr. Fung Yat-kong and staff of the Hong Kong University Press are gratefully acknowledged.

We are also very much grateful to the Lee Wing Tat Fund for Education and Research in Medicine for financial support for this publication.

Organizing Committee

T.K. Chan (Chairman)
Vivian Chan
S.K. Lam
W.K. Lam
Christina Wang
Y.L. Yu

CONTRIBUTORS

Professors:

Chan, T.K., MD, FRCP (Edin), FRCP (Lond) 　陳棣光
Lam, S.K., MD, FRCP (Edin), FRCP (Lond) 　林兆鑫
Wang, Christina C.L., MD, FRACP, FRCP (Glas) 　汪重輪
Young, Rosie T.T., OBE, MD, FRCP (Edin), FRCP (Glas), FRCP (Lond), FRACP, JP 　楊紫芝

Readers:

Chan, Vivian N.Y., MSc, PhD, DIC, FACB 　陳立怡
Kumana, C.R., BSC, MB BS, FRCP (Can), FRCP (Lond)
Lai, C.L., MB BS, FRCP (Edin), FRCP (Lond) 　黎青龍
Lam, W.K., MD, FRCP (Edin) 　林華杰
Yu, Y.L., MD, FRCP (Edin) 　余毓靈

Senior Lecturers:

Lam, Karen S.L., MB BS, MRCP (UK) 　林小玲
Lok, Anna S.F.. MB BS, MRCP (UK) 　駱淑芳

Lecturers:

Chang, P.C.M., MB BS, MRCP (UK) 　張茲勘
Cheng, C.H., MB BS, MRCP (UK) 　鄭俊豪
Cheng, I.K.P., MB BS, PhD, FRACP 　鄭鑑波
Chiu, E.K.W., MB BS, MRCP (UK) 　趙健華
Ip, Mary S.M., MB BS, MRCP (UK) 　葉秀文
Kung, Annie W.C., MB BS, MRCP (UK) 　龔慧慈
Lau, C.P., MB BS, MRCP (UK) 　劉柱柏
Liang, R.H.S., MB BS, MRCP (UK) 　梁憲孫
Pun, K.K., MD, MRCP (UK) 　潘建基
Tai, Y.T., MB BS, MRCP (UK) 　戴有鼎
Wong, K.L., MB BS, MRCP (UK), FRACP 　黃基林

Honorary Clinical Lecturers:

Cheung, K.L., MB ChB, FRCP (Edin) (Consultant Cardiologist, University Medical
　Unit, Grantham Hospital) 　張敬瓏
Hui, W.M., MB BS, MRCP (UK) (Senior Medical Officer, University Medical Unit,
　Tung Wah Hospital) 　許偉武

TRIBUTE AND BIOGRAPHY

David Todd (達安輝)

OBE, JP, AM(Hon), MD, FRCP, FRCP (Edin), FRCP (Glas), FRACP

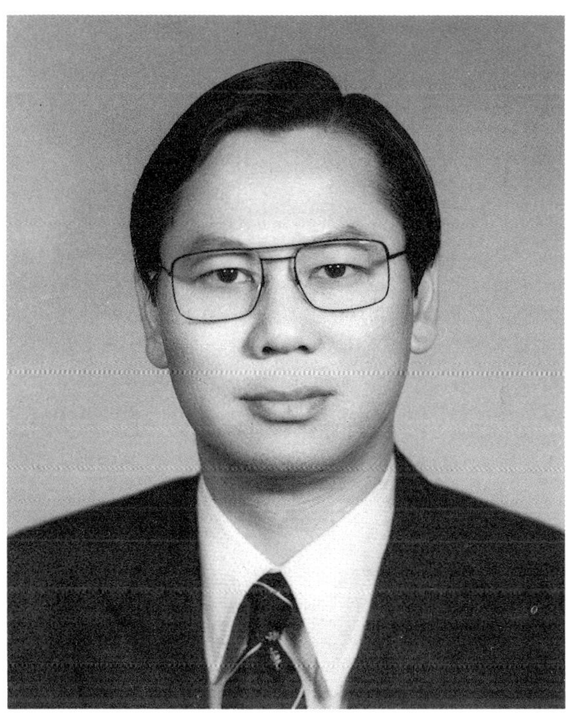

David Todd was born 61 years ago, in the year of the dragon (1928), in Canton, nowadays Guangzhou. His adopted parents were missionaries from United States and his father, Dr. Paul J. Todd, started the Kung Yee Hospital, one of the first medical schools in Canton, which later became the Chung Shan University Medical School. Subsequently, the Todd Clinic and Hospital was built and served the region until this was taken over in 1949 by the Chinese Government and renamed the Second People's Children Hospital. In 1980, when we were both invited to lecture at Chung Shan Medical School, he brought me to the Hospital and pointed out fondly the building opposite the Outpatient Department, where he spent his childhood; and, I am sure, where he inculcated the idea of becoming a medical practitioner to serve the poor and the needy. He went to primary school at True Light School and when Canton fell

to the Japanese, he came to Hong Kong and attended Diocesan Boys' School as a boarder. With the Winds of World War II he went into free China to study at Lingnan Middle School which had moved inland to Ku Kong (Shaoguan County). After the war he returned to the city of his birth as freshman in Lingnan University Medical School. A second change of fortune brought him to the University of Hong Kong in 1947, to complete his undergraduate training. This has proven to be a great loss to Guangzhou but an enormous gain for Hong Kong.

In the University, he excelled in all undergraduate subjects: was awarded the two Ho Fook and Chan Kai Ming Prizes for first place in the second and final MB examinations, as well as the Ng Li Hing Prize in Anatomy and Ho Kam Tong Prize in Public Health. After completing the then newly introduced house physician year, he was appointed full time teaching staff in the University Department of Medicine at Queen Mary Hospital in 1953. Except for two years (1956–1958) as Sino-British Fellow and Honorary Registrar at the Muirhead Department of Medicine, Royal Infirmary Glasgow, Scotland, he has remained with the University. He obtained MRCP (Edinburgh) in 1957 and MD (HK) in 1958. He rose in position from Senior Clinical Assistant to Assistant Lecturer (1955), Lecturer (1958), Senior Lecturer (1964), Reader (1966) to the first Personal Professorship in Medicine in 1972. When Professor AJS McFadzean retired in 1974, he became Professor of Medicine and Head of the Department.

He taught and trained generations of medical practitioners and was chosen by the students as Best Teacher at the only time this award was given in the University. He is a great proponent of postgraduate and continued education. He firmly believes and practises what Osler said about medical education that it '. . . is not a college course, not a medical course but a life course for which the work of a few years under teachers is but a preparation . . .' for life-long self education.

He has been Overseas Examiner for MRCP(UK) since 1980 and it is mainly a credit to his negotiation and persuasion that the MRCP examination can now be completed in Hong Kong — the only overseas centre to have gained this salutatory status. He founded the Hong Kong College of Physicians in 1986 and has been its President since. The Singapore Academy of Medicine awarded an AM(Hon) to him in 1986 for contributions to postgraduate teaching in the National University. Within the Department, he established the AJS McFadzean Library and has been largely responsible for updating the books, monographs and journals which induced and enticed senior and junior staff alike to continued self education. His breadth and depth of knowledge on recent advances has always astounded the staff and he is a storehouse of new and important information.

His contact with North American Medicine started with a Travelling Fellowship awarded by China Medical Board in 1964. He returned as Research Fellow to the Department of Human Genetics, University of Michigan in 1970 and Visiting Research Haematologist at UCSF in 1973. In turn, the K.P Stephen Chang and Mr and Mrs Wu Chung Visiting Professorships in Medicine, established by him in the Department, has allowed many prominent physicians from USA and other countries to visit Hong Kong and participate in teaching and discussions in research, with great benefits to students and staff. The Tai Ping Shan Visiting Professorship, the Tam Ho Kit Ching Visiting Professorship in Nephrology and the AJS McFadzean Lecturership have also achieved their purposes with visitors from U.K., Australia, Canada and USA. Professor Maxwell M Wintrobe in his book 'Hematology, the Blossoming of a Science: a Story of Inspiration and Effort.' wrote about David Todd: 'Alex McFadzean's successor as Professor of Medicine . . . began studies in hematology by investigating polycythemia in primary cancer of the liver and inquiring into the pathogenesis of cryptogenetic splenomegaly. He then went on to study molecular genetics and population characteristics of G6PD deficiency and thalassemia in his part of the world where he now is one of the leading hematologists.'

His Australasia contact has also been prolific, following a long period of exchanges during the McFadzean years. He was appointed Councillor of RACP 1980–1986 — a singular honour for a person outside Australia. He is indeed a man of many continents which he treads with sincerity and in a gentlemanly fashion which has been recognized as distinctively David Todd. When presenting him for admission as Honorary Academician in the Singapore Academy of Medicine, Dr. P.H. Feng cited that 'In spite of his many academic and professional achievements David nevertheless has remained essentially an unassuming and unpretentious individual. ... His analytical mind, incisive intellect, quiet manner, and compassion for his fellow man epitomizes the best from both East and West and make him what he is — a gentleman extraordinaire. If there had been no David Todd to light up the path of Medicine in this region, it would have been necessary to invent him.'

Besides playing the international arena and putting Hong Kong on the map, he has also contributed to local medical and educational institutions. He was Subdean of the Medical Faculty (1976–1978), Pro-Vice-Chancellor (1978–1980) and member of UPGC (since 1986). He was member of Medical Development Advisory Committee (1977–1987), Vice-Chairman of the Hong Kong Kidney Foundation, Vice-President of Federation of Medical Societies (1975–1977). His vast experience and knowledge in medical matters made him the ideal person to be appointed recently to the Committee on Management and Funding of Teaching Hospitals, which is of crucial importance for the future of the University's clinical departments. We are relieved that David will be there to advise and help to steer the new Hospital Authority in the right direction. For his immense contribution to medical affairs in Hong Kong, the Queen conferred on him the Most Excellent Order of Officer of the British Empire in 1982.

Amidst this high profile and public commitments, David never loses sight of his priorities as a clinician and an academic. He continued ward rounds in general medical and special haematology wards, attended outpatients both to heal and to teach. He maintained a keen interest in haematology/oncology research and kept up to date with recent advances in patient care in all medical subspecialties. His list of original publications numbered over 100. His accomplishments in thalassemia, malignant lymphoma and chronic liver diseases will be reviewed in the respective section in this symposium. He was awarded the Carl de Gruchy Medal of the Haematology Society of Australia in 1979. He has been visiting professor, external examiners in many University and was internal examiner for 30 MDs.

Under his headship, all subspecialties were given a free hand to develop, if he was not paving the way, he would be assisting in the background. His *'laissez-faire'* policy, famous for Hong Kong's economic success, has also been very successful here as evidenced by the achievements in each subspecialty. This is particularly remarkable considering the limited support from the University and Government during this period. He once remarked to me that his philosophy is to allow and encourage free enterprise and his role is to lean in one or the other direction. For the unsuccessful 'entrepreneur', the inevitable outcome of despair and frustration occurred. However, for the majority of those who left the Department, they had developed most successfully and were in their prime to seek fame and fortune in other positions. He always kept contact with these past staff members and gave his wise counsel freely. Professor YW Kan wrote when he received the Lita Annenberg Award for excellence in clinical research in 1984: 'A number of events have been pivotal in formulating my career. Through the encouragement of David Todd, I decided to take up hematology and come to America'. Y.W. is still collaborating with David on thalassaemia research. The 1997 problems have created unrest in Hong Kong and has resulted in an increased rate of resignation of our well qualified physicians. David held the helm unwaivingly and maintained the high standard of clinical service in the Department. We are glad that he has accepted the Vice-Chancellor's offer to remain in the Department as a stabilizing force and to provide his wise counsels on University and Medical matters.

In conclusion, David Todd is an accomplished academician, a practising physician of the highest calibre, an administrator, a skilful politician and a irreplaceable Head for the Department of Medicine. The staff of the department has gathered here today to honour him and to review the achievements in his Department from 1974 to 1989.

T.K. CHAN

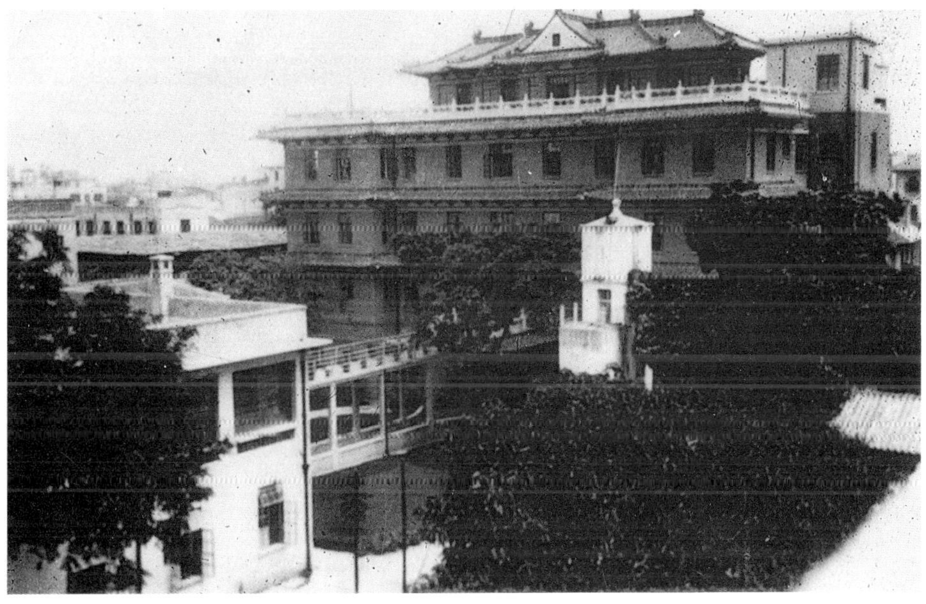

Todd Clinic & Hospital, Guangzhou, China, 1928

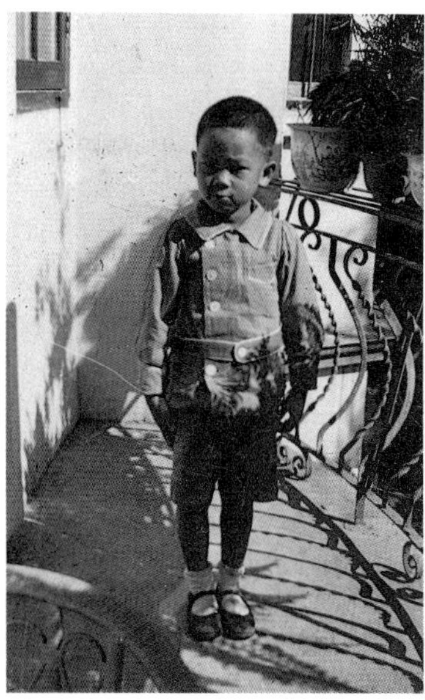

On the verandah of the resident wing of the Todd Clinic & Hospital

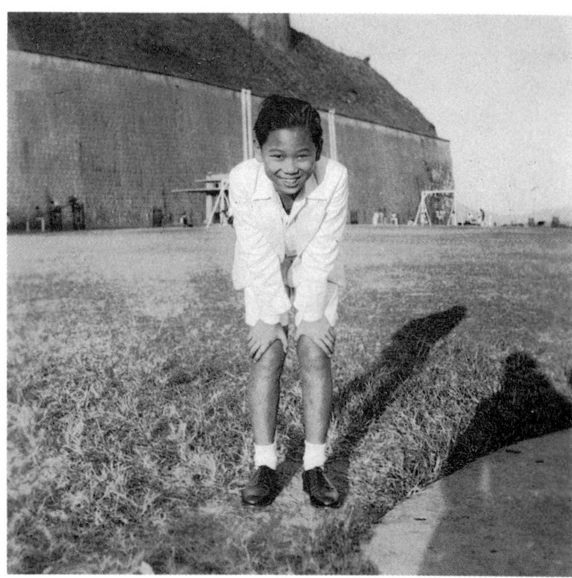

As a boarder in Diocesan Boys' School, with Kowloon Observatory in background

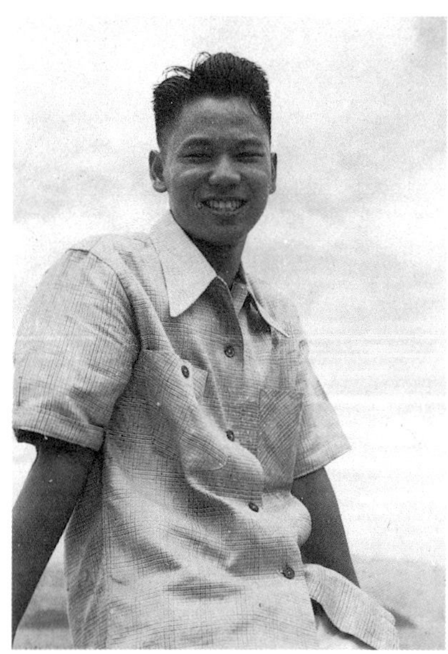

At Lingnan Middle School

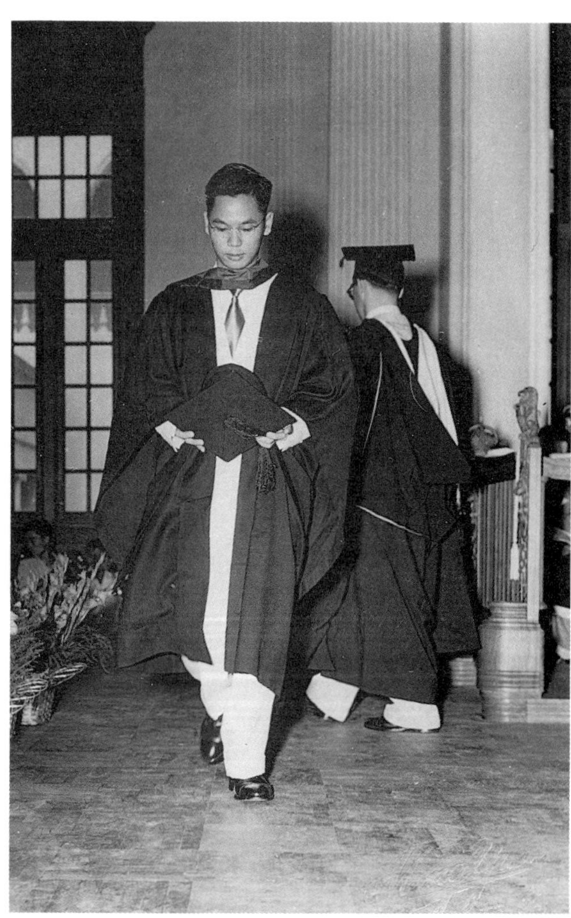

MB,BS (HK), 1952

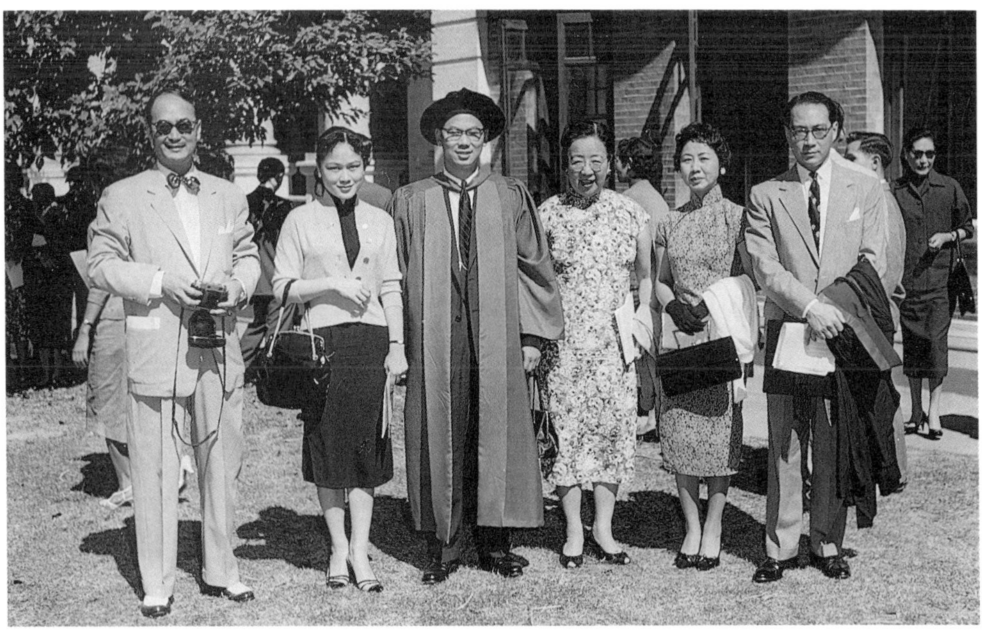

MD (HK), 1958

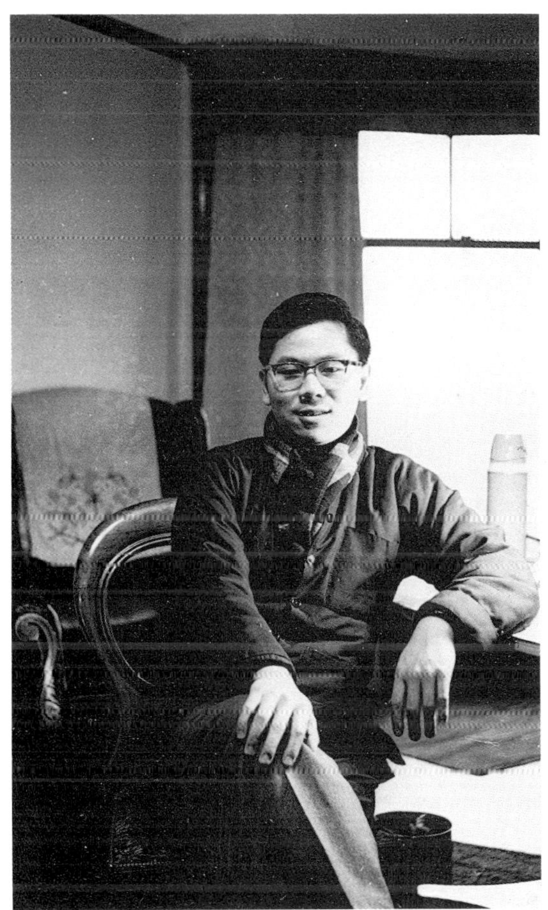

Sino-British Fellow in Glasgow, U.K., 1957

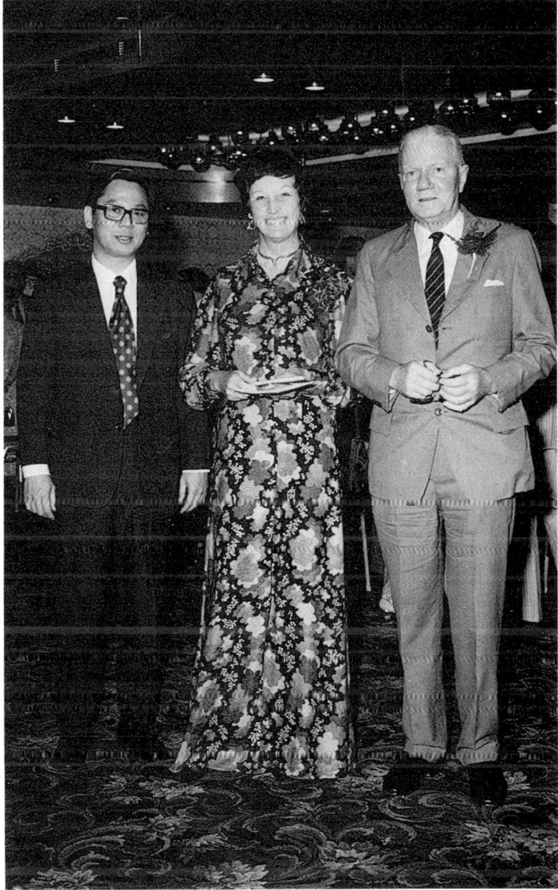

With Professor and Mrs. A.J.S. McFadzean, 1974

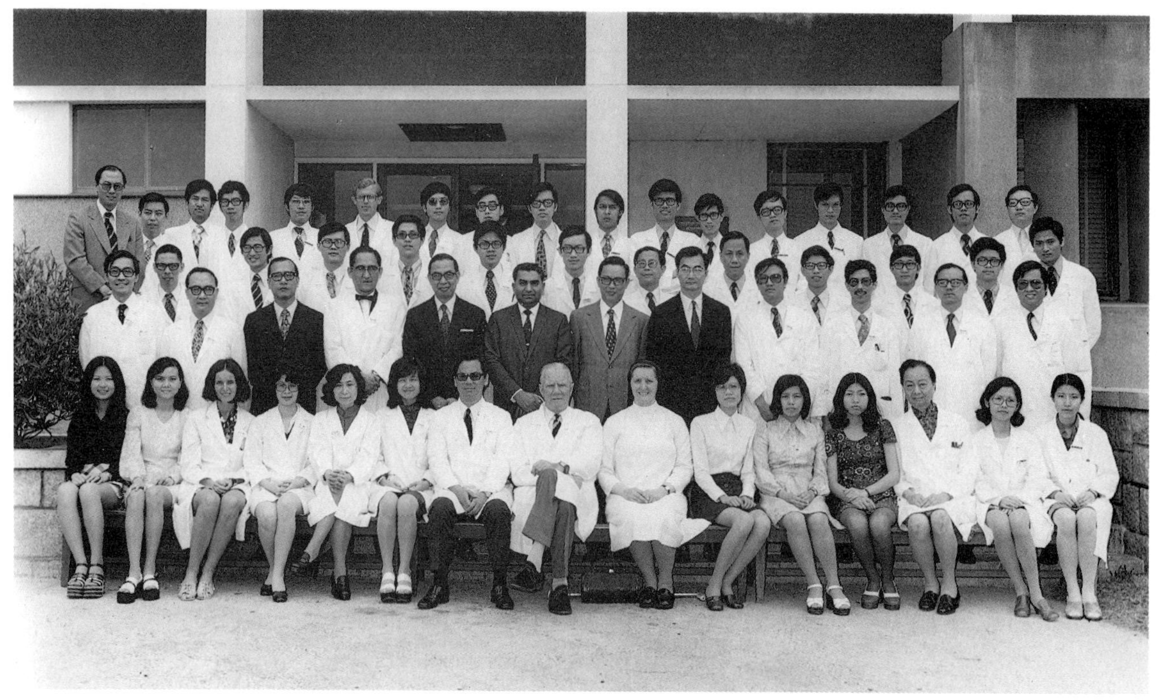

Department of Medicine, University of Hong Kong, 1974

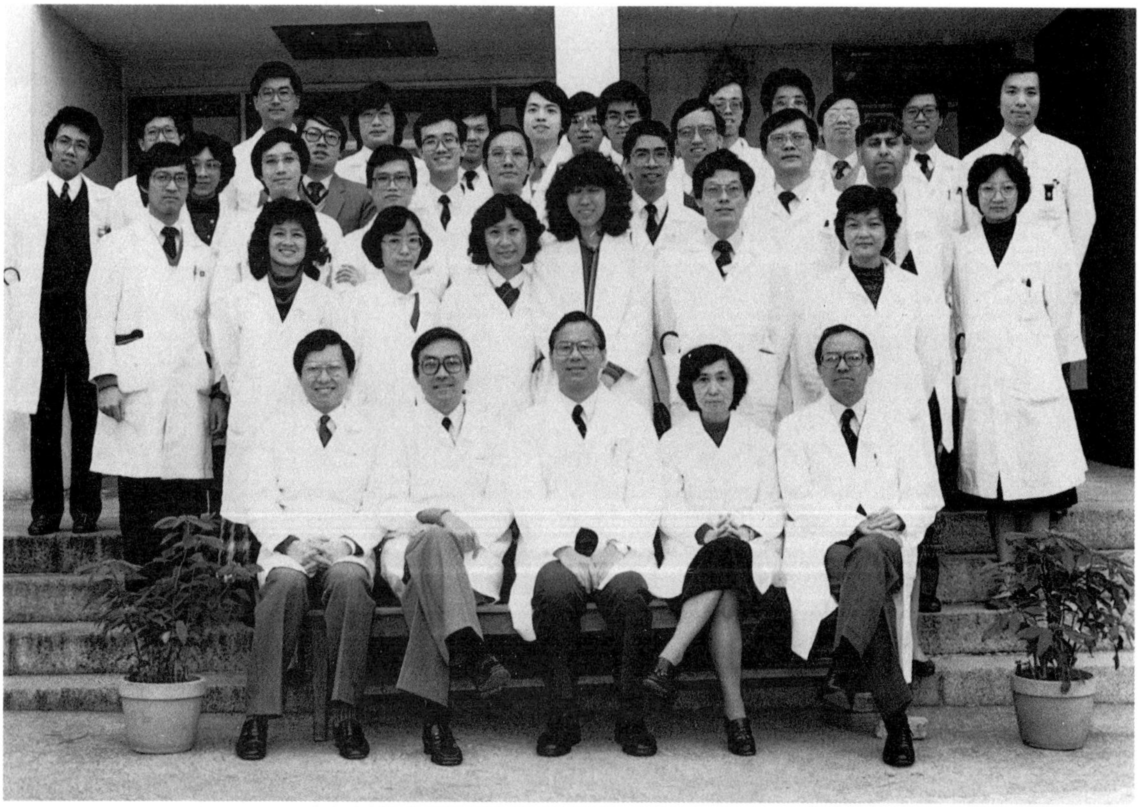

Department of Medicine, University of Hong Kong, 1985

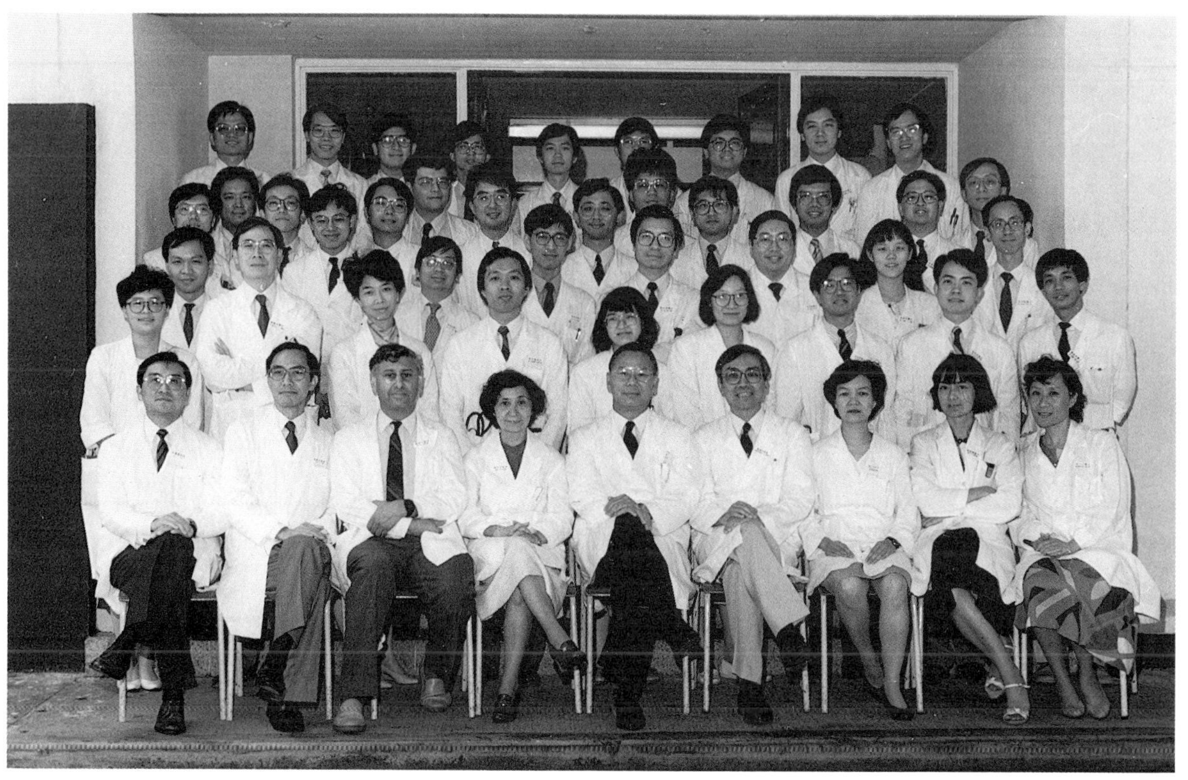

Medical staff of the Department of Medicine, University of Hong Kong, 1989

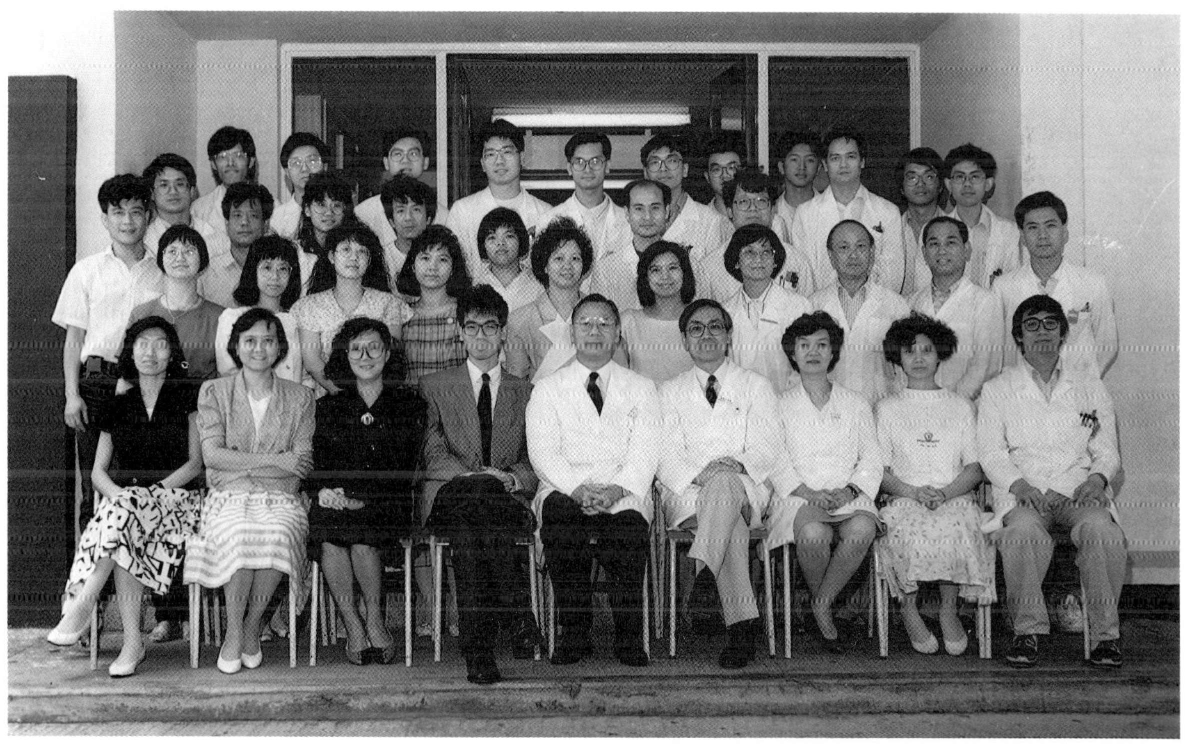

Other staff of the Department of Medicine, University of Hong Kong, 1989

Curriculum Vitae of Professor David Todd

Date of Birth: November 17th, 1928

Marital Status: Unmarried

Medical Qualifications

M.B., B.S. (H.K.)	1952
M.D. (H.K.)	1956
Royal College of Physicians of Edinburgh, Member	1957
Royal College of Physicians of Edinburgh, Fellow	1966
Royal Australasian College of Physicians, Fellow	1974
Royal College of Physicians of London, Member	1975
Royal College of Physicians of London, Fellow	1976
Royal College of Physicians and Surgeons of Glasgow, Fellow	1979

Honours

Unofficial Justice of Peace	1977
O.B.E.	1982
A.M. (Hon.), Academy of Medicine Singapore	1986

Education

Secondary School: Diocesan Boys' School, Hong Kong, and Lingnan University Middle School, Ku Kong, China.

Lingnan University Medical School, Canton: 1945–1947 (transferred to University of Hong Kong in 1947)

University of Hong Kong, Faculty of Medicine: 1947–1952

Prizes

Ho Fook and Chan Kai Ming Prize in Anatomy and Physiology (awarded co-equally), University of Hong Kong, May 1949.

Ng Li Hing Prize in Anatomy, University of Hong Kong, May 1949.

Ho Kam Tong Prize in Public Health, University of Hong Kong, May 1951.

Ho Fook and Chan Kai Ming Prize in Medicine, Surgery and Obstetrics & Gynaecology (awarded co-equally), University of Hong Kong, May 1952.

Appointments

July 1952–June 1953: House Physician, University Department of Medicine, Queen Mary Hospital, Hong Kong.

Since July 1953: Full-time teaching staff of the University of Hong Kong, Department of Medicine, Queen Mary Hospital, Hong Kong.

1953/1954	Senior Clinical Assistant
1955–1958	Assistant Lecturer
1958–1964	Lecturer
1964–1966	Senior Lecturer
1966–1972	Reader
1972–1974	Personal Professorship
1974–1989	Professor of Medicine & Head of Department
1989–	Professor of Medicine

Other Appointments

1974–1989: Consultant in Medicine, Government of Hong Kong.

1975–1985: Honorary Consultant in Medicine to the British Army in Hong Kong.

1976/1978: Sub-Dean, Faculty of Medicine, University of Hong Kong.

1978/1980: Pro-Vice-Chancellor, University of Hong Kong.

Internal Examiner of M.D. Candidates

1975	Dr. LAM Shiu Kum
1977	Dr. YIP Shing Kwan
1978	Dr. NG Kah Wai, Thomas
1979	Dr. HSU Lee Keung, George
1980	Dr. CHAN LUI Wai Ying
	Dr. TENG Chong Shing
	Dr. WONG Kwok On
1981	Dr. YU Yu Hei, Victor
1982	Dr. CHAN Man Kam
	Dr. LEE Sum Ping
	Dr. YU Yu Chiu, Donald
1983	Dr. CHAN Tai Kwong
	Dr. CHEN Wai Chee, Walter
	Dr. HO Chi Suk, Faith
	Dr. LAI Kai Neng
	Dr. WANG Yu Ching, Rebecca
1984	Dr. WU Pui Chee
1985	Dr. YU Yuk Ling
1986	Dr. LAM Wah Kit
1987	Dr. PUN Kin Kee
	Dr. YEUNG Choi Kit
1988	Dr. CHAN Wing Chung
	Dr. LAM Tai Hing
	Dr. LAM Tak Sum
	Dr. TANG Chang Hung, Lawrence
1989	Dr. LAU Chu Pak
	Dr. WOO Kam Sang

Overseas Postgraduate Activities

1956/1958: Sino-British Research Fellow, The Sino-British Fellowship Trust, and Honorary Registrar at the Muirhead Department of Medicine, University of Glasgow, Royal Infirmary, Glasgow.

January/June 1964: Travelling Fellow, China Medical Board of New York Inc. visiting various departments of medicine in the U.S.A.

May/June 1967: Visiting Lecturer, Department of Haematology, University College Hospital Medical School, London, England.

September/December 1970: Research Fellow, Department of Human Genetics, University of Michigan, Michigan, U.S.A.

September/December 1973: Visiting Research Haematologist, Department of Medicine, University of California Medical School, San Francisco, California, U.S.A.

October/November 1974: Visiting Professor, Academy of Medicine, Singapore.

March 1978: Norman Paul Visiting Professor, Sydney Hospital, Sydney, Australia.

August 1979: Carl de Gruchy Lecturer, Haematology Society of Australia, Australia.

April 1982: Visiting Lecturer in Haematology, National University of Singapore, Singapore.

1980 to present: Overseas Examiner for the M.R.C.P.(U.K.) Part II Examination, Royal Colleges of Physicians of the United Kingdom.

External Examiner in Medicine:
University of Tasmania (1975)
National University of Singapore (1980 & 1986)
National University of Malaysia (1983)

Short visits to medical centres in the U.K., U.S.A., Australia and S.E. Asia, often to lecture, and attendances at international and regional conferences are not included.

Membership of Learned Societies

International Society of Haematology — Asian Pacific Division, 1972–
Association of Physicians of Great Britain and Ireland, 1973–
International Association for the Study of the Liver, 1974–1985
Hong Kong Biochemical Association, 1978–
American Association for the Advancement of Science, 1972–
New York Academy of Science, 1981–
British Blood Transfusion Society, 1984–

Medals

Long Service Medal, Auxiliary Medical Service, Hong Kong.

Membership of Public Bodies and Committees

I.   UNIVERSITY OF HONG KONG
Court, Senate and Board of the Faculty of Medicine and various sub-committees.

II.   OUTSIDE OF THE UNIVERSITY OF HONG KONG
1. Honorary Consultant in Medicine, Hong Kong Government, 1974–1989.
2. Honorary Consultant in Medicine, British Army in Hong Kong, 1975–1985.
3. Member, Medical Development Advisory Committee, 1977–1987.
4. Member, Medical Subcommittee, University & Polytechnic Grants Committee, Hong Kong Government, 1984–1987.
5. Member, University & Polytechnic Grants Committee, Hong Kong Government, 1986–1991.
6. Chairman, Research Subcommittee, University & Polytechnic Grants Committee, Hong Kong Government, 1987–
7. Chief Examiner in Medicine, Licentiate Examination (Pt. I) of the Medical Council of Hong Kong, 1976–1986.
8. Chief Examiner in Medicine, Licentiate Examination (Pt. III) of the Medical Council of Hong Kong, 1976–1984.
9. Director, Hong Kong Tuberculosis, Chest & Heart Diseases Association, 1973–1989.
10. Member, Grantham Hospital Management Committee, 1973–1989.
11. Vice-Chairman, Hong Kong Kidney Foundation Limited, 1979–
12. Member and Past Chairman, Hong Kong Society of Haematology, 1972–
13. Censor, Hong Kong College of General Practitioners, 1978–1988.
14. President, Hong Kong College of Physicians, 1986–
15. President, Hong Kong Society of Antimicrobial Chemotherapy, 1988–1989.
16. Chief Censor, Hong Kong College of General Practitioners, 1986–1988.
17. Member, Lingnan College Council, 1983–1985.
18. Vice-President, Hong Kong Sino-British Fellowship Trust Scholars' Association, 1982–
19. Member, Sino-British Fellowship Trust Selection Committee, 1976–
20. Member, Selection Committee of the Croucher Foundation, 1982–
21. Honorary Adviser, Hong Kong Medical Technologists Association, 1975–
22. Honorary Adviser, St. James' Settlement, 1974–
23. Overseas Adviser (Hong Kong), Royal College of Physicians, London, 1979–
24. Adviser, Royal College of Physicians & Surgeons of Glasgow, 1984–
25. Council Member, Royal Australasian College of Physicians, 1980–1986.
26. Examiner, Examiners' Panel, Royal College of Physicians of the U.K., 1980–
27. MRCP(UK) Examination Board: Examiner and Organizer for Hong Kong 1985–
28. Assessor, National Health and Medical Research Council of Australia Project Grant Scheme, 1977–
29. Honorary Adviser, Roche Far East Research Foundation, 1972–
30. Representative for Hong Kong, Ciba Foundation, London, 1983–
31. Member of Editorial Board, Medical Progress, 1973–1984.
32. Member of Editorial Board, Medicine Digest (South-East Asian edition), 1983–1984.
33. Member, Branch Committee, Hong Kong Red Cross, March 1975–April 1977.
34. Member, Management Board, Blood Transfusion Service, Hong Kong Red Cross, January 1975–September 1978.
35. Vice-President, Federation of Medical Societies of Hong Kong, 1975–1977.
36. Chairman, Working Party on the Scadding/Fox Report on 'Tuberculosis in Hong Kong : Present position and future planning of methods of control and treatment' (Medical and Health Department and Hong Kong Anti-Tuberculosis & Thoracic Diseases Association), 1975/1976.
37. Committee Member, Royal Commonwealth Society, Hong Kong Branch, 1982–1984.
38. Editorial Director, Journal of American Medical Association — Southeast Asian Edition, 1984–
39. Assessor, Anti-Cancer Council of Victoria, Australia, 1986–
40. Member, International Advisory Com-

mittee, Journal of the American Medical Association, 1987–

41. Medical & Health Department, Hong Kong Government:
    Member, Advisory Committee on Hepatitis B Vaccination
    Member, Advisory Committee on Acquired Immune Deficiency Syndrome
    Member, Ethical Committee

42. Member, Committee on Management and Funding of Teaching Hospitals, Provisional Hospital Authority, 1989 —

Publications

1. McFadzean AJS, **Todd D**, Tsang KC: Polycythaemia in primary carcinoma of the liver. *Blood* 1958; 13: 427.

2. McFadzean AJS, **Todd D**, Tsang KC: Observations on the anaemia of cryptogenetic splenomegaly. I. Haemolysis. *Blood* 1958; 13: 513.

3. McFadzean AJS, **Todd D**, Tsang KC: Observations on the anaemia of cryptogenetic splenomegaly. II. Expansion of plasma volume. *Blood* 1958; 13: 524.

4. **Todd D**: Observations on the aminoaciduria in megaloblastic anaemia. *J Clin Path* 1959; 12: 238.

5. **Todd D**: Ascorbic acid deficiency in Addisonian Pernicious Anaemia. *Scot Med J* 1959; 4: 249.

6. Kan YW, McFadzean AJS, Tso SC, **Todd D**: Further observations on polycythaemia in hepatocellular carcinoma. *Blood* 1961; 18: 592.

7. Cook J, McFadzean AJS, **Todd D**: Splenectomy in cryptogenetic splenomegaly. *Brit Med J* 1963; 2: 337.

8. Chan TK, **Todd D**, Wong CC: Erythrocyte glucose-6-phosphate dehydrogenase deficiency in Chinese. *Brit Med J* 1964; 2: 102.

9. McFarlane, AS, **Todd D**, Cromwell S: Fibrinogen catabolism in humans. *Clin Sci* 1964; 26: 415.

10. McFadzean AJS, **Todd D**: The distribution of Cooley's anaemia in China. *Trans Roy Soc Trop Med Hyg* 1964; 58: 490.

11. **Todd D**, Kan PS: Anaemia in prengnancy in Hong Kong. *J Obstet Gynaec Brit Cwlth* 1976; 72: 738.

12. Chan TK, **Todd D**, Wong CC: Tissue enzyme levels in erythrocyte glucose-6-phosphate dehydrogenase deficiency. *J Lab Clin Med* 1965; 66: 937.

13. Chan TK, **Todd D**, Wong CC: Erythrocyte glucose-6-phosphate dehydrogenase activity in haemoglobin H disease. *Nature* 1966; 209: 1147.

14. McFadzean AJS, **Todd D**: The blood volume in post-necrotic cirrhosis of the liver with splenomegaly. *Clin Sci* 1967; 32: 339.

15. McFadzean AJS, **Todd D**, Tso SC: Erythrocytosis associated with hepatocellular carcinoma. *Blood* 1967; 29: 808.

16. **Todd D**, Lai M, Braga CA: Thalassaemia and Hydrops Foetalis — family studies. *Brit Med J* 1967; 3: 347.

17. Irvine WJ, McFadzean AJS, **Todd D**, Tso SC, Young RTT: Pernicious Anaemia in the Chinese: a clinical and immunological study. *Clin & Exper Immunology* 1969; 4: 375.

18. **Todd D**, Lai MCS, Braga CA, Soo HN: Alpha thalassaemia in Chinese: cord blood studies. *Brit J Haemat* 1969; 16: 551.

19. McCurdy PR, Blackwell RQ, **Todd D**, Tso SC, Tuchinda S: Further studies on G-6-PD deficiency in Chinese subjects. *J Lab & Clin Med* 1970; 75: 788.

20. **Todd D**, Lai MCS, Beaven GH, Huehns ER: The abnormal haemoglobins in homozygous alpha-thalassaemia. *Brit J Haemat* 1970; 19: 27.

21 Chan TK, Chesterman CN, McFadzean AJS, **Todd D**: The survival of glucose-6-phosphate dehydrogenase-deficient erythrocytes in patients with typhoid fever on chloramphenicol therapy. *J Lab & Clin Med* 1971; 77: 177.

22. Kwan CS, **Todd D**: The Clinical significance of occasional red-cells with haemoglobin H inclusions. *J Hong Kong Med Tech Assoc* 1971; 1: 7.

23. McFadzean AJS, **Todd D**: Cooley's Anaemia among the Tanka of South China. *Trans Roy Soc Trop Med Hyg* 1971; 65: 59.

24. Chan TK, **Todd D**, Lai MCS: Glucose-6-phosphate dehydrogenase: identity of erythrocyte and leukocyte enzyme with report of a new variant in Chinese. *Biochem Genet* 1972; 6: 119.

25. Chan TK, **Todd D**: Characteristics and distribution of glucose-6-phosphate dehydrogenase-deficient variants in South China. *Amer J Hum Genet* 1972; 24: 475.

26. Fessas P, Lie-Injo LE, Na-Nakorn S, **Todd D**, Clegg JB, Weatherall DJ: Identification of slow-moving haemoglobins in haemoglobin H disease from different racial groups. *Lancet* 1972; 1: 1308.

27. So PL, Chan TK, Lam SK, Teng CS, Young RTT, **Todd D**: Cortisol metabolism in glucose-6-phosphate dehydrogenase deficiency. *Metabolism* 1973; 22: 1443.

28. Kan YW, **Todd D**, Dozy AM: Haemoglobin constant spring synthesis in red cell precursors. *Brit J Haemat* 1974; 28: 103.

29. Taylor JM, Dozy AM, Kan YW, Varmus HE, Lie-Injo LE, Ganesan J, **Todd D**: Genetic lesion in homozygous α-thalassaemia (Hydrops Fetalis). *Nature* 1974; 251: 392.

30. Kan YW, **Todd D**, Holland JP, Dozy AM: Absence of α-globin mRNA in homozygous α-thalassaemia. *J Clin Invest* 1974; 53: 37a.

31. **Todd D**: Diagnosis of haemolytic states. *Clinics in Haematology* 1975; 4: 63.

32. Chan TK, **Todd D**: Haemolysis complicating viral hepatitis in patients with glucose-6-phosphate dehydrogenase deficiency. *Brit Med J* 1975; l: 131.

33. Kan YW, Dozy AM, Varmus HE, Taylor JM, Holland JP, Lie-Injo LE, Ganesan J, **Todd D**: Deletion of α-globin genes in haemoglobin H disease demonstrates multiple α-globin structural loci. *Nature* 1975; 255: 255.

34. Kan YW, Taylor JM, Dozy AM, Varmus HE, Lie-Injo LE, Ganesan J, **Todd D**: Homozygous α-thalassemia (Hydrops Fetalis): evidence for deletion of the structural gene. In: *Erythrocyte Structure and Function* (ed. GJ Brewer), AR Liss, New York, 1975; p. 139.

35. Chan TK, **Todd D**, Tso SC: Drug induced haemolysis in glucose-6-phosphate dehydrogenase deficiency. *Brit Med J* 1976; 2: 1227.

36. **Todd D**: Physician training in Hong Kong. *Chronicle* (Royal College of Physicians, Edinburgh) 1976; 6: 14.

37. Kan YW, Dozy AM, Trecantin RF, **Todd D**: Identification of a non-deletion type of α-thalassemia defect. *Blood* 1976; 48: 999.

38. Chan WC, Lai KS, **Todd D**: Adult Niemann-Pick Disease — A case report. *J Path* 1977; 121: 177.

39. Ng RP, **Todd D**: Management of malignant lymphomas: a brief review. *Bull Hong Kong Med Assoc* 1977; 29: 13–20.

40. Tso SC, Chan TK, **Todd D**: Aplastic anaemia: a study of prognosis and the effect of androgen therapy. *Q J Med* 1977; 46(184): 513–529.

41. Kan YW, Dozy AM, Trecartin R, **Todd D**: Identification of a non-deletion defect in α-thalassemia. *New Eng J Med* 1977; 297: 1081–1083.

42. Dozy AM, Kabisch H, Baker J, Koenig HM, Kurachi S, Stamatoyannopoulos G, **Todd D**, Kan YW: The molecular defects of α-thalassemia in the Filipino. *Hemoglobin* 1977; 1: 539–546.

43. Ho FCS, **Todd D**: Malignant histiocytosis. Report of five Chinese patients. *Cancer* 1978; 42(5): 2450–2460.

44. **Todd D**, Chan TK: Hemoglobin Bart's levels in umbilical cord blood: failure as a method for distinguishing mild from severe α-thalassemia trait in the Chinese. *Hemoglobin* 1978; 2(4): 389–392.

45. Lam SK, Wong KP, Chan PKW, Ngan H, **Todd D**, Ong GB: Fatal cholangitis after endoscopic retrograde cholangiopancreatography in congenital hepatic fibrosis. *Aust NZ J Surgery* 1978; 48(2): 199–202.

46. Wong V, Ma HK, **Todd D**, Golbus MS, Dozy AM, Kan YW: Diagnosis of homozygous α-thalassemia in cultured amniotic-fluid fibroblasts. *N Engl J Med* 1978; 298: 669–670.

47. Lam KC, Lai CL, Wu PC, **Todd D**: Etiological spectrum of liver cirrhosis in the Chinese. *J Chronic Dis* 1979; 33: 375–381.

48. Lai CL, Wu PC, Lam KC, **Todd D**: Histologic prognostic indicators in hepatocellular carcinoma. *Cancer* 1979; 44(5): 1677–1683.

49. Lie-Injo LE, Dozy AM, Kan YW, Lopes M, **Todd D**: The α-globin gene adjacent to the gene for Hb Q-α[74 Asp-His] is deleted, but not that adjacent to the gene for Hb G-α[30 Glu-Gln]; three-fourths of the α-globin genes are deleted in HbQ-α-thalassaemia. *Blood* 1979; 54, 6: 1407–1416.

50. Chan V, Chan TK, Wong V, Tso SC, **Todd D**: The determination of antithrombin III by radioimmunoassay and its clinical

application. *Brit J Haemat* 1979; 41: 563–572.

51. **Todd D**: Thalassaemia and haemoglobinopathies. *Medicine* 1980; 27: 1406–1412.

52. Ko RC, Wong FWT, **Todd D**, Lam KC: Prevalence of Toxoplasma Gondii antibodies in the Chinese population of Hong Kong. *Trans Roy Soc Trop Med Hyg* 1980; 74(3): 351–354.

53. Wang C, Ng RP, Chan TK, **Todd D**: Effect of combination chemotherapy on pituitary-gonadal function in patients with lymphoma and leukemia. *Cancer* 1980; 45(8): 2030–2037.

54. Tso SC, **Todd D**: Anaemias and their management in Southeast Asia. *Medical Progress* 1980; 7: 13–22.

55. Tso SC, Wong V, Chan V, Chan TK, Ma HK, **Todd D**: Deep vein thrombosis and changes in coagulation and fibrinolysis after gynaecological operations in Chinese: the effect of oral contraceptives and malignant disease. *Brit J Haemat* 1980; 46: 603–612.

56. **Todd D**, Chan V, Schneider RG, Dozy AM, Kan YW, Chan TK: Globin chain synthesis in Haemoglobin New York (β113 Valine → Glutamic acid). *Brit J Haemat* 1980; 46: 557–564.

57. Embury SH, Miller JA, Dozy AM, Kan YW, Chan V, **Todd D**: Two different molecular organizations account for the single α-globin gene of the α-thalassemia-2 genotype. *J Clin Invest* 1980; 66: 1319–1325.

58. Lai CL, Lam KC, Wong KP, Wu PC, **Todd D**: Clinical Features of hepatocellular carcinoma : review of 211 patients in Hong Kong. *Cancer* 1981; 47: 2746–2755.

59. **Todd D**: Postgraduate medical education in Hong Kong. *Proceedings of the Royal College of Physicians of Edinburgh, Tercentenary Congress, 1981* (ed. R Passmore), pp. 333–338.

60. Li AMC, Lee FT, **Todd D**: The screening of Chinese cord blood for haemoglobinopathies. *Human Heredity* 1982; 32: 62–70.

61. Wong V, Chan TK, Chan V, Tso SC, **Todd D**, Ma HK: The effect of oral contraceptives on coagulation and fibrinolytic parameters in the Chinese : a prospective study. *Thrombosis & Haemostasis* 1982; 48(3).

62. Lai CL, Lam KC, Wong KP, Wu PC, **Todd D**: Clinical features of hepatocellular carcinoma. *Oncology Digest, International Synopses* 1982; 1: 12.

63. Ng RP, **Todd D**, Khoo RKK: Salvage chemotherapy for non-Hodgkin's lymphoma. *Cancer Treatment Reports* 1982; 66(11): 1977–1979.

64. Tso SC, Chan TK, **Todd D**: Venous thrombosis in haemoglobin H disease after splenectomy. *Aust NZ J Med* 1982; 12(6): 635–638.

65. Aquinas M, **Todd D**: Particular problems of tuberculosis in developing countries. In: *Oxford Textbook of Medicine* (eds. DJ Weatherall, JGG Ledingham, DA Warrell), Oxford University Press, Oxford, 1983; 1: 5.262–5.266.

66. **Todd D**: Haematologic disorders in Southeast Asia. *Medical Progress Special Issue* 1983; pp. 69–72.

67. Kumana CR, Ng M, Lin HS, Ko W, Wu PC, **Todd D**: Hepatic veno-occlusive disease due to toxic alkaloid in herbal tea. *Lancet* 2 1983; 1361.

68. **Todd D**: Invited review : thalassaemia. *Pathology* 1984; 16(1): 5–15, 19.

69. Tso SC, Loh TT, **Todd D**: Iron overload in patients with haemoglobin H disease. *Scand J Haemat* 1984; 32: 391, 394.

70. Chan V, Ghosh A, Chan TK, Wong V, **Todd D**: Prenatal diagnosis of homozygous α thalassaemia by direct DNA analysis of uncultured amniotic fluid cells. *Brit Med J* 1984; 288: 1327–1329.

71. Lai CL, Wu PC, Yeoh EK, Lok ASF, Lin HJ, Lam SK, **Todd D**: Hepatocellular carcinoma and the hepatitis B virus. In: *Viral Hepatitis B Infection in the Western Pacific Region: Vaccine and Control,* Singapore World Scientific Publications Co., 1984; pp. 3 16.

72. Chan V, Leung NK, Chan TK, Ghosh A, Kan YW, **Todd D**: BamH I polymorphism in the Chinese: its potential usefulness in prenatal diagnosis of β thalassaemia. *Brit Med J* 1984; 289: 947–948.

73. Ho FCS, **Todd D**, Loke SL, Ng RP, Khoo RKK: Clinico-pathological features of malignant lymphomas in 294 Hong Kong Chinese patients. Retrospective study covering an eight-year period. *Int J Cancer* 1984; 34: 143–148.

74. Kumana CR, Ng M, Lin HJ, Ko W, Wu PC, **Todd D**: Herbal tea induced hepatic veno-

occlusive disease: quantification of toxic alkaloid exposure in adults. *Gut* 1985; 26: 101–104.

75. Chin D, Tse TM, Wong WS, **Todd D**, Yu CP, Mann KS: Paraparesis with hemoglobin E-β thalassemia. *Aust NZ J Med* 1985; 15: 263–264.

76. Liang ST, Wong VCW, So WWK, Ma HK, Chan V, **Todd D**: Homozygous α-thalassaemia: clinical presentation, diagnosis and management. A review of 46 cases. *Brit J Obst & Gynae* 1985; 92: 680–684.

77. Chan V, Chan TK, Liang ST, Ghosh A, Kan YW, **Todd D**: Hydrops fetalis due to an unusual form of Hb H disease. *Blood* 1985; 66(1): 224–228.

78. Chan V, Chan TK, Cheng MY, Leung NK, Kan YW, **Todd D**: Characteristics and distribution of β thalassaemia haplotypes in South China. *Human Genetics* 1986; 73: 23–26.

79. Chan V, Chan TK, Cheng MY, Kan YW, **Todd D**: Organization of the ζ-α genes in Chinese. *Brit J Haemat* 1986; 64: 97–105.

80. Ho FCS, Loke SL, Hui PK, **Todd D**: Immunohistological subtypes of non-Hodgkin's lymphoma in Hong Kong Chinese. *Pathology* 1986; 18: 426–430.

81. Kumana CR, Chau PY, **Todd D**: How should we use cephalosporins. *The Hong Kong Practitioner* 1986; 8(12): 2183–2186.

82. Woo E, Yu YL, Ng M, Huang CY, **Todd D**: Spinal cord compression in multiple myeloma: who gets it? *Aust NZ J Med* 1986; 16: 671–675.

83. Woo E, Yue CP, Mann KS, Cheung FMF, Chan TK, **Todd D**: Intracerebral chloromas. Report of a case and review of the literature. *Clin Neurol Neurosurg* 1986; 88–2: 135–139.

84. Liang R, **Todd D**, Chan TK, Wong KL, Ho F, Loke SL: Peripheral T cell lymphoma. *J Clin Oncology* 1987; 5(5): 750–755.

85. Chan V, Chan TK, Tso SC, **Todd D**: Combination of three α-globin gene loci deletions and hemoglobin New York results in a severe hemoglobin H syndrome. *Am J Hemat* 1987; 24: 301–306.

86. Aquinas M, **Todd D**: Particular problems of tuberculosis in developing countries. In: Oxford Textbook of Medicine, 2nd edition (eds. DJ Weatherall, JGG Ledingham, DA Warrell), Oxford University Press, Oxford,

1987; 1: 5.299–5.303.

87. **Todd D**: Continuing medical education. *Annals of Academy of Medicine, Singapore* 1987; 16(2): 366–369.

88. Liang R, **Todd D**: Current management of non-Hodgkin's lymphoma. *Medical Progress* 1987: 17–28.

89. Liang R, Ng RP, **Todd D**, Choy D, Khoo RKK, Ho FCS: Management of stage I–II diffuse aggressive non-Hodgkin's lymphoma of the Waldeyer's Ring: combined modality therapy versus radiotherapy alone. *Haemat Oncol* 1987; 5: 223–230.

90. **Todd D**, Kumana CR, So SY, Cheng IKP, Wong KL, Chan CW, Chiu W, Chow E, Chu KM: Clinical pathological conference. A patient with chronic renal failure and lung shadow. *J HK Med Assn* 1987; 39(2): 109–114.

91. Chan V, Chan TK, Ghosh A, Wong LC, Ma HK, Kan YW, **Todd D**: Application of DNA polymorphisms for prenatal diagnosis of β thalassemia in Chinese. *Amer J Hemat* 1987; 25: 409–415.

92. Chan V, Chan TK, Chebab FF, **Todd D**: Distribution of β thalassemia mutations in South China and their association with haplotypes. *Amer J Hum Genet* 1987; 41: 678–685.

93. Liang RHS, **Todd D**, Chan TK, Ho FCS, Ng RP: Gastrointestinal lymphoma in Chinese: a retrospective analysis. *Hemat Oncol* 1987; 5: 115–126.

94. Liang R, **Todd D**, Chan TK, Ng RP, Choy D, Loke SL, Ho FSC: Follicular non-Hodgkin's lymphoma in Hong Kong Chinese: a retrospective analysis. *Hemat Oncol* 1988; 6: 29–37.

95. Liang R, Chan TK, **Todd D**: Chemotherapy for relapsed and resistant acute nonlymphoblastic leukemia. *Cancer Chemother Pharmacol* 1988; 21: 68–70.

96. Chan V, Chan TK, Wong ACK, Chan TPT, Ghosh A, **Todd D**: Restriction fragment length polymorphism in the interzeta hypervariable region for prenatal diagnosis of nondeletion α thalassemia. *Amer J Haemat* 1988; 27: 242–246.

97. Chan V, Chan TK, **Todd D**: Prenatal diagnosis of homozygous α thalassemia 1 (hemoglobin Barts hydrops fetalis). In: *Prenatal Diagnosis of Thalassemia and the Hemo-*

globinopathies (ed. Loukopoulos D), CRC Press, Inc., Florida, USA, 1988; Chapter 16, pp. 209–220.

98. Chan TK, Chan V, **Todd D**, Ghosh A, Wong LC, Ma HK: Prenatal diagnosis of α-and β-thalassemias: experience in Hong Kong. *Hemoglobin* 1988; 12(5 & 6): 787–794.

99. Chan V, Chan TK, Kan YW, **Todd D**: A novel β-thalassemia frameshift mutation (Codon 14/15), detectable by direct visualization of abnormal restriction fragment in amplified genomic DNA. *Blood* 1988; 72: 4: 1420–1423.

100. Chan V, Chan TK, **Todd D**: Different forms of Hb H disease in the Chinese. *Hemoglobin* 1988; 12(5 & 6): 499–507.

101. Liang R, Yung RWH, Chau PY, Chan TK, Lam WK, So SY, **Todd D**: Imipenem/cilastatin as initial therapy for febrile neutropenic patients. *J Antimicrob Chemother* 1988; 22(6): 765–770.

102. Liang R, **Todd D**, Chan TK: HOAP-Bleo as salvage therapy for diffuse aggresive non-Hodgkin's lymphoma. *Cancer Chemother Pharmacol* 1988; 22(2): 169–172.

103. Liang R, Woo EKW, Yu YL, **Todd D**, Chan TK, Ho FCS, Tso SC, Shum JST: Central nervous system involvement in non-Hodgkin's lymphoma. *Eur. J. Cancer Clin Oncol* 1989; 25(4): 703–710.

104. Liang R, Chan TK, Chan GTC, **Todd D**: Treatment of adult acute lymphoblastic leukaemia using an intensive chemotherapy protocol. *Cancer Chemother Pharmacol* 1989; 23(6): 384–388.

105. Cheng PNM, Tso SC, Chan TK, **Todd D**, Lawton JWM, Ho FCS: Acute lymphoblastic leukemia in Chinese adults in Hong Kong. *Aust NZ J Med* 1989; 19: 37–43.

106. Chan EYT, Chan GTC, **Todd D**, Ho FCS, Pi D: Peripheral T cell lymphoma presenting as haemophagocytic syndrome. *Hematol Oncol* 1989; 7: 275.

107. Wang C, Tso SC, **Todd D**: Hypogonadotropic hypogonadism in severe b-thalassemia: effect of chelation and pulsatile gonadotropin-releasing hormone therapy. *J Clin Endocrinol Metab* 1989; 68(3): 511–516.

108. Liang R, Choi P, **Todd D**, Chan TK, Choy D, Ho F: Hodgkin's disease in Hong Kong Chinese. *Hematol Oncol* 1989 (in press).

109. Lau JYN, Lai CL, Lin HJ, Lok ASF, Liang RHS, Wu PC, Chan TK, **Todd D**: Fatal reactivation of chronic hepatitis B virus infection following chemotherapy withdrawal in lymphoma patients. *Q J Med* 1989 (in press).

110. Liang R, Yung RWH, Chan TK, Chau PY, Lam WK, So SY, **Todd D**: Ofloxacin versus co-trimoxazole for prevention of infection in neutropenic patients. *Antimicrob Agents and Chemother* 1989 (in press).

111. Chan V, Chan TK, Tong TMF, **Todd D**: A novel missense mutation in exon 4 of the factor VIII: C gene resulting in moderately severe Hemophilia A. *Blood* 1989 (in press).

Abstracts

1. McFadzean AJS, **Todd D**: Anaemia in post-necrotic cirrhosis of the liver with splenomegaly. *XIth Congress of the International Society of Haematology, 1966, Abstracts*; p. 149.

2. **Todd D**: Family studies of hydrops foetalis with haemoglobin Bart's. *XIth Congress of the International Society of Haematology, 1966, Abstracts*; p. 269.

3. **Todd D**, Chan TK, Tso SC: Red-cell survival in glucose-6-phosphate dehydrogenase deficiency. *Proceedings of XIIIth International Congress of Haematology, August 2–8, 1970*, Lehmanns Verlag, Munchen; p.180.

4. **Todd D**, Kan YW, Dozy AM: Hemoglobin constant spring: possibly unstable messenger-RNA and evidence for the two loci therapy for alpha-chain production. *Clin Res* 1972; 20: 471.

5. **Todd D**, Kan YW, Dozy AM: Globin-chain synthesis in various alpha-thalassemia syndromes. *XIV International Congress of Hematology, Sao Paulo, Brazil, July 16–21, 1972, Abstracts*; p. V.

6. Kan YW, Dozy AM, Varmus HE, Taylor JM, Holland JP, Lie-Injo LE, Ganesan J, **Todd D**: The Molecular basis of the α-thalassaemia syndromes. *Clin Res* 1975; 23: 398.

7. **Todd D**: α-thalassaemia in Chinese. *Proceedings, III Meeting of Asian Pacific Division, International Society of Haematology, Jakarta, 1975*.

8. Chan TK, **Todd D**: Can xylitol infusion pre-

vent oxidative haemolysis in G6PD deficiency? *Proceedings, III Meeting of the European and African Division, International Society of Haematology, London, 1975.*

9. **Todd D**, Dozy AM, Kan YW, Golbus MS: The molecular defects of the α-thalassaemia syndromes. *XVI International Congress of Hematology, Kyoto, 1976, Abstracts*; p. 54

10. Tso SC, Chan TK, **Todd D**: Prognosis and conventional therapy in aplastic anaemia. *XVI International Congress of Hematology, Kyoto, 1976, Abstracts*; p. 78.

11. **Todd D**, Ho FCS, Khoo RKK: Malignant lymphoma in Chinese. *XVI International Congress of Hematology, Kyoto, 1976*; p. 205.

12. Tso SC, Chan TK, **Todd D**: The spleen in haemoglobin H disease. *XVII Congress of International Society of Hematology, Paris, 1978, Abstracts*; 1: 371.

13. Wang C, Ng RP, **Todd D**: Effect of combination chemotherapy on pituitary-gonadal function in patients with malignant lymphoma. *XVII Congress of International Society of Hematology, Paris, 1978, Abstracts*; 2: 890.

14. **Todd D**, Chan V, Chan TK: Globin-chain synthesis in a family with haemoglobin New York. *XVII Congress of the International Society of Hematology, Paris, 1978, Abstracts*; 1: 323.

15. Ng RP, **Todd D**, Khoo RKK, Ho FCS: Combination chemotherapy in non-Hodgkin's lymphoma. *Annual Meeting, Haematology Society of Australia and Australian Society of Blood Transfusion, Hobart, 1979, Abstract.*

16. **Todd D**: Alpha-thalassaemia. *Annual Meeting, Haematology Society of Australia and Australian Society of Blood Transfusion, Hobart, 1979, Abstract*; p. 293.

18. **Todd D**: Haemoglobin constant spring and human haemoglobin synthesis. *Fourth Meeting of Asian Pacific Division, International Society of Haematology, Seoul, Korea, June 25–29, 1979, Abstract*; p. 17.

19. **Todd D**, Chan V, Tso SC, Chan TK: Haemoglobinopathies in the Chinese. *Fourth Meeting of Asian Pacific Division, International Society of Haematology, Seoul, Korea, June 25–29, 1979, Abstract*; p. 77.

20. Ng RP, **Todd D**, Ho FCS, Khoo RKK: Histiocytic diffuse non-Hodgkin's lymphoma. *Fourth Meeting of Asian Pacific Division, International Society of Haematology, Seoul, Korea, June 25–29, 1979, Abstract*; p. 42.

21. Ng RP, **Todd D**: Prednisone, cytosine arabinoside & CCNU (PAC)-salvage chemotherapy for non-Hodgkin's lymphoma. *Proceedings of the International Society of Blood Transfusion, Budapest, Hungary, August 1982, Abstract*; p. 171.

22. Tso SC, Loh TT, **Todd D**: Iron status in thalassaemia syndromes. *Proceedings of 19th Congress of International Society of Haematology and 17th Congress of International Society of Blood Transfusion, Budapest, Hungary, August 1982, Abstract*; p. 218.

23. Ho FCS, Tso SC, **Todd D**: Splenic Histology in chronic idiopathic thrombocytopenia — correlation with clinical outcome. *Proceedings of 19th Congress of International Society of Haematology and 17th Congress of International Society of Blood Transfusion, Budapest, Hungary, August 1982, Abstract*, p. 353.

24. **Todd D**, Chan VNY: Haemoglobin H disease in Chinese. *Proceedings of the Fifth Meeting of the Asian-Pacific Division of the International Society of Haematology, Manila, January 1983, Abstract*; p. 6.

25. Ng RP, Ho Wat FCS, Khoo RKK, **Todd D**: Waldeyer's ring non-Hodgkin's lymphoma (with Ng RP, Ho Wat Faith CS, Khoo RKK). *Proceedings of the Fifth Meeting of the Asian-Pacific Division of International Society of Haematology, Manila, January 1983, Abstract*, p. 9.

26. Chan V, Chan TK, **Todd D**: Different ζ-α gene organisation in the Chinese. *International Conference on Thalassaemia, Bangkok, 1985, Abstract*; p. 39.

27. Chan V, Chan TK, Liang ST, Ghosh A, Kan YW, **Todd D**: Hydrops fetalis due to an unusual form of Hb H disease. *International Conference on Thalassaemia, Bangkok, 1985, Abstract*; p. 66.

28. Chan VNY, Chan TK, **Todd D**: Molecular heterogeneity of Hb H disease in the Chinese. *The Twenty-first Congress of the International Society of Haematology, Sydney. Oral Presentation Tu 1–7, May 1986, Abstract*; p. 300.

29. Chan VNY, Chan TK, Cheng MY, Leung NK, Kan YW, **Todd D**: Beta-thalassaemia haplotypes in the Chinese. *The Twenty-first*

Congress of the International Society of Haematology, Sydney. Oral Presentation Tu 1–3, May 1986, Abstract; p. 299.

30. **Todd D**, Chan V, Chan TK: Haemoglobinopathies/thalassaemia in Southern Chinese (with Chan V, Chan TK). *XXI Congress of I.S.H., Sydney, May 1986, Abstract, Symposium*; M4–5, p. 120.

31. **Todd D**, Chan V, Chan TK, Ghosh A, Liang ST, Ma HK: Antenatal diagnosis of α-thalassaemia. *XXI Congress of I.S.H., Sydney, May 1986, Abstract, Symposium*; Tu 3–3, p. 149.

32. Liang R, Chan TK, **Todd D**: Chemotherapy for relapsed and resistant acute non-lymphoblastic leukaemia-effect of ATA, an amsacrine containing regime. *4th International Symposium on Therapy of Acute Leukaemia, Feb. 1987, Abstract*; p. 575.

33. Liang R, **Todd D**, Chan TK, Wong KL, Ho F, Loke SL: Peripheral T cell lymphoma. *3rd International Conference on Malignant Lymphoma, June 1987, Abstract*; p. 16.

34. Liang R, Ng RP, **Todd D**, Chan TK, Choy D, Khoo RKK, Ho FCS: Management of stage I–II diffuse aggressive non-Hodgkin's lymphoma of the Waldeyer's ring: combined modality therapy versus radiotherapy alone. *4th European Conference on Clinical Oncology, Nov. 1987, Abstract*; p. 990.

35. Choi P, Liang R, Choy D, **Todd D**: Hodgkin's disease — A Hong Kong experience. *The Royal College of Radiologists' Annual Meeting, Sept. 1988.*

36. Liang R, Chiu E, Yung R, Chau PY, Chan TK, Lam WK, So SY, **Todd D**: Imipenem/cilastatin for febrile neutropenic infection. *The 4th European Congress of Clinical Microbiology, April 1989.*

37. Liang R, Chan V, Chan TK, **Todd D**, Ho F, Choi P: Gene rearrangement of peripheral blood and bone marrow: lymphoma of mucosa-associated lymphoid tissue. *The 25th Annual Meeting of the American Society of Clinical Oncology, San Francisco, U.S.A. May, 1989, Abstract*; p. 1014.

38. Liang R, Yung R, Chan TK, Chau PY, Lam WK, So SY, **Todd D**: Ofloxacin versus co-trimoxazole for prevention of infection in neutropenic patients following cytotoxic chemotherapy. *The 29th Interscience Conference on Antimicrobial Agents and Chemotherapy, Sept. 1989, Abstract*; p. 316.

Letters

1. Smith JB, **Todd D**: Foetal globin in primary liver cancer. *Lancet* 1968; 2: 833.

2. **Todd D**: Slow-moving haemoglobin bands in haemoglobin H disease. *Lancet* 1971; 2: 439.

3. Ng RP, Chan TK, **Todd D**: The Nitro-blue Tetrazolium Test: false negatives and false positives. *Lancet* 1972; 1: 1341.

4. Wang C, Ng RP, Chan TK, **Todd D**: Leydig cell dysfunction after combination chemotherapy. *Lancet* 1981; 2: 529 (Letter to Editor).

5. Ho Wat FCS, Chan GTC, **Todd D**: Non-specificity of sudan black B in the diagnosis of acute myeloid leukaemia. *Brit J Haemat* 1983; 53(1): 171–172.

Editorials

1. **Todd D**, Tso SC: Treatment of aplastic anaemia. *Medical Progress* (Editorial) 1974; 1: 15.

2. **Todd D**: Treatment of common anaemias. *Medical Progress* (Editorial) 1974; 1: 16.

3. Tso SC, **Todd D**: Treatment of aplastic anaemia. *Medical Progress* (Editorial) 1974; 1: 15.

4. **Todd D**: Thalassaemia: current concepts in management. *Medical Progress* (Editorial) 1976; 3: 17.

5. **Todd D**: Southeast Asia and JAMA. *JAMA SEA* (Editorial) Jan 1985; p. 5.

6. **Todd D**: Contempo '85. *JAMA SEA Contempo* (Editorial) 1985; p. 5.

7. **Todd D**: The Economic impact of the acquired immune deficiency syndrome. *JAMA SEA* (Editorial) April 1986; p. 5.

8. **Todd D**: Continuing medical education. *JAMA SEA* (Editorial) Jan 1987; p. 5.

9. **Todd D**: Molecular biology and clinical medicine. *JAMA SEA* (Editorial) Jan 1989; p. 4.

ACHIEVEMENTS IN CARDIOLOGY

Division of Cardiology in Queen Marry Hospital

The cardiac division is an active unit offering increasing services to our local community. It has kept up with advances in various aspects of cardiology, thus maintaining its leading role amongst the government and subvented hospitals in Hong Kong. Since 1974, the cardiac division has been served by the following physicians: Dr. Victor Yan, Dr. T.F. Tse, Dr. Rebecca Wang, Dr. Walter Chen, Dr. P.K. Lee, Dr. Philip Wong, Dr. Joseph Chow, Dr. K.K. Hui, Dr. Y.T. Tai, Dr. C.P. Lau and myself.

In the span of 15 years (1974–1989), the division can view with pride the progressively better care it offers to patients with cardiac disorders. It began with only two clinics, those of general cardiology and hypertension. Today, the division is responsible for eight clinics, namely hypertension, general cardiac, echocardiogram, pacemaker, arrhythmia, valvular, post percutaneous coronary angioplasty (post-PTCA) and post balloon valvuloplasty clinics. The addition of these special clinics ensures better care for these subsets of patients who require close monitoring by doctors trained in the respective fields.

The 'up-grading' of the cardiac catheterization laboratory (Lewis Laboratory) in Queen Mary Hospital by Dr. T.F. Tse and Dr. Rebecca Wang has enabled us to perform coronary angiogram, vital in the management of patient with ischaemic heart disease.

Since the introduction of electrophysiology study (E.P.S.) by Dr. Rebecca Wang in 1980, the number of cases the division handles also increases with years. In the recent two years, Dr. Y.T. Tai & Dr. C.P. Lau perform these investigations on a regular basis. Since the introduction of echocardiography and cardiac exercise laboratory by Dr. T.F. Tse in 1976, we are now performing five to six thousands echocardiograms per year.

In the recent few years, the introduction of intervention cardiology has proven to be of great help in the management of certain cardiac diseases. Dr. Rebecca Wang performed the first coronary angioplasty. Dr. K.L. Cheung and myself introduced the technique of percutaneous balloon mitral and pulmonary valvuloplasty into this department in 1988. Dr. C.P. Lau performed the 1st electrical ablation of the AV node.

The cardiac division, because of its progressively more advanced technology, extended technical skill and professional expertise, has become the referral centre for complicated cardiac problems from other regional hospitals:Princess Margaret Hospital, United Christian Hospital, Kwong Wah Hospital, Caritas Medical Centre and Nethersole Hospital.

The statistical figures in Table 1 provides a picture of the various kind of cases the division has dealt with.

In addition to the tremendous service workload in the ward and clinic, the physicians in the division have to take up undergraduate teaching and supervise postgraduate training in clinical cardiology as well as basic techniques in cardiac investigation like echocardiography, pacing and cardiac catheterization. They also shared in the general medical ward duties of the Department.

Research

Research activities have not been slighted and most of the academic pursuits are clinically orientated. These are reviewed in the following subheadings.

Haemodynamic Evaluation of Drugs for Heart Failure

Systematic study of various drugs in the treatment of heart failure (26, 27, 31, 49, 50, 52).

Recently, β adrenoreceptor downgrading has been considered to be an important aggravating cause in worsening heart failure. The use of β-blocker in such situation may be beneficial. Labetalol, an agent with combined α & β blocking

Table 1. Activities of Lewis Laboratory at Queen Mary Hospital 1974 to 1989

Year	Cardiac Catheterization	Coronary Angiography	Temporary Pacing	Permanent Pacing	E.P.S.	Echocardio-graph	Holter Monitor
1974	127	6	26	23	0		
1975	225	12	35	26	0		
1976	280	16	42	4	0		
1977	366	44	50	42	0		
1978	366	60	33	46	0	1080	
1979	393	64	32	48	0	1682	47
1980	347	92	65	75	18	1252	115
1981	317	107	94	13	17	283	
1982	290	77	80	43	11	984	309
1983	319	98	90	69	7	2292	448
1984	364	133	97	73	15	5447	646
1985	223	82	72	40	4	8020	700
1986	298	184	78	40	0	6731	969
1987	180	77	70	40	0	6530	1060
1988	223	117	109	74	94	5169	1067
1989 (Aug)	228	191	57	51	77	2049	976

activity, was used in the treatment of dilated cardiomyopathy (114).

Coronary Artery Disease

The epidemiology study of acute myocardial infarction is well recognised in Caucasian population but it is controversial whether this could be applied to the predominantly Chinese population in Hong Kong. From June 1985 to April 1988, 325 consecutive cases of acute myocardial infarction admitted to the University Medical Unit in Queen Mary Hospital were prospectively studied for the in-hospital course and risk factors (60). Coronary anatomy was studied in Chinese patients with ischaemic heart disease (22, 34).

Cardiac Catheterization and Echocardiogram

Technique in performing cardiac catheterization in patients with aortic valve stenosis and the justification of caridac catheterization before valvular replacement were discussed (36, 75). Non invasive echocardiographic assessment of patient with different kinds of artificial valves,

and organic valvular disease were also discussed (32, 48, 58, 61, 62, 82, 88).

Mitral Valve Prolapse

A systemic analysis of the prevalence of mitral valve prolapse in Chinese and its associated skeletal abnormalities were reviewed (72, 73, 74, 76).

Antihypertensive Treatment

Various kind of antihypertensive drugs have been tried in our department before its introduction to the local community (56).

Cardiac Arrhythmia Management

Although digoxin is the classical treatment for atrial fibrillation, it is less effective in controlling the rate during exercise and excitement. Other nodal slowing agents may improve this, yet they require time to act and do not improve regularity. A new pacing method by inserting a paced ventricular beat after a conducted beat in atrial fibrillation was devised, which is termed intercalated pacing (140).

Various antiarrhythmic drugs have been tried to assess their efficacy in the management of ventricular tachycardia (40).

Electrical ablation of the AV node was also performed in the management of refractory arrhythmia (119).

Atrial Natriuretic Peptide

Atrial natriuretic peptide was measured, as a collaborating work with the medical department in Chinese University, in patients with giant atrium (113), and in patients with a variety of pacing modalities.

Rate Responsive Pacing

Pacemakers, which are capable of adjusting the rate in time of needs, have been shown to be beneficial both haemodynamically and functionally. Study was performed on different sensors (minute ventilation and body movement sensing). Our centre is the first in South East Asia to implant minute ventilation, temperature sensing, and dual chamber rate response pacemakers (99, 104, 106).

Observation Studies

Our heavy clinical involvement is reflected in the large number of clinical observations we have made. This includes congenital heart disease, acquired heart disease, cardiac pacing and arrhythmia (55, 59, 65, 69, 78, 87, 90, 91, 96 97, 100–103, 105, 108–117, 121, 126, 127).

Cyanotic Congenital Heart Disease

Patients with Eisenmenger complex have a poor prognosis. A study was carried out to assess the effect of oral nifedipine in relieving the reversible component of pulmonary hypertension (98). The value of two-dimensional echocardiography was discussed (37).

Pregnancy in Patients with Prosthetic Heart Valve

The incidence and the type of anticoagulant used during pregnancy were studied (35, 47, 63, 67).

Prosthetic Valve and Antiplatelet Agent

The effect of antiplatelet agents on patients with prosthetic valves was studied (42, 64, 68).

Local Journals

Many articles were written on various topics in cardiology in local cardiac and general practitioner's journals (2–8, 10–13, 24, 28–30, 41, 92, 118–120, 129).

All these achievements were made possible with the leadership of the Head of department, Professor Todd and the team of dedicated physicians working literally day and night.

Publications

1. Yan V: Pericarditis in acute myocardial infarction. *Heart Lung* 1974; 3 (2): 247.
2. Yan V: Beta adrenergic receptor blocking agents. *Proc HK Cardiol Soc* 1974; 1 (1): 2.
3. Yan V: Electrocardiogram in cor pulmonale. *Proc HK Cardiol Soc* 1974; 1 (1): 19.
4. Yan V: Sick sinus node syndrome. *Proc HK Cardiol Soc* 1974; 1 (1): 29.
5. Yan V: The use of beta-blocking agent in Hong Kong. In: *Advances in Beta-adrenergic Blocking Therapy. Proceedings of an International Symposium* (ed. Snart AG), Excerpta Medica, Amsterdam, 1974; 4: 86.
6. Yan V: Diagnosis of rheumatic fever. *Proc Hk Cardiol Soc* 1974: 1 (2): 72.
7. Yan V: Ventricular arrhythmias. *Proc HK Cardiol Soc* 1975; 2 (1): 39.
8. Yan V: Myocardial ischaemia. *Proc HK Cardiol Soc* 1975; 2 (1): 59.
9. Yan VWT: Editorials: Treatment of angina. *Med Prog* 1975; 2 (3): 17.
10. Yan V: Permanent cardiac pacing in Hong Kong. *Proc HK Cardiol Soc* 1975; 2 (2): 105.

11. Yan V: Long term drug therapy in hypertension. *Proc HK Cardiol Soc* 1975; 2 (2): 125.

12. Yan V: Exercise electrocardiogram. *Proc HK Cardiol Soc* 1976; 3 (1): 17.

13. Yan V: Clinical approach to patients with cardiac arthythmias. *Proc HK Cardiol Soc* 1977; 4: 7.

14. Yan V, Hunt D, Sloman G: Double blind study of corticosteroid therapy in the management of pericardial pain in acute myocardial infarction. *Aust NZ J Med* 1973; 3: 101.

15. Yan V: Pericarditis. In: *Coronary Care Workbook*, 2nd edition (eds. Hunt D, Sloman G), Australasian Drug Information Services Pty Limited, 1973; p. 78.

16. Yan V: Dissecting aortic aneurysm. In: *Coronary Care Workbook*, 2nd edition (eds. Hunt D, Sloman G), Australasian Drug Information Services Pty Limited, 1973; p. 166.

17. Yan V, Sloman G: Clinical value of the telephono-transmitted electrocardiogram. *Med J Aust* 1973 (special suppl); 2: 33.

18. Vohra J, Hunt D, Yan V, Sloman G: Sick sinus node syndrome. *Med J Aust* 1973 (special suppl); 2: 41.

19. Yan V, Sloman G: Double blind cross over study of the inotropic influence of tiprenolol (DU 21445) and propranolol in patients with ischaemic heart disease. *Aust NZ J Med* 1973; 3: 467.

20. Tse TF, Wang R, Ng R: Diagnosis of acute rheumatic fever and infective endocarditis. *Phil J Internal Medicine* 1977; 15: 103–110.

21. Wang R, Camm J, Ward D, Washington H, Martin A: The assessment of drug treatment of atrial fibrillation in the elderly. In: The Proceedings of the 3rd International Symposium on Ambulatory Monitoring 1979 (eds. Stott FD, Rafterey EB, Goulding L), Academic Press, London; pp. 113–120.

22. Wang RYC, Chen WWC, Lee PK: Preliminary report on coronary artery disease as documented by coronary angiography among Chinese in Hong Kong. *Proc HK Cardiol Soc* 1979; 6: 207–209.

23. Ward DE, Camm AJ, Wang R, Dymond D, Spurrell RAF: Suppression of long-standing incessant ventricular tachycardia by amiodarone. *J Electrocardiol* 1980; 13: 193–198.

24. Wang R: The current concepts on the use of digitalis. *Bull HK Med Assoc* 1980; 32: 33–36.

25. Woo E, Wang R, Lai CL: Fatal aminopyrine-induced pancytopenia. *Bull HK Med Assoc* 1980; 32: 29–31.

26. Wang RYC, Lee PK, Yu DYC, Tse TF, Choiw MSS: Haemodynamic and myocardial metabolic effects of terbutaline in severe heart failure. *Am J Cardiol* 1981; 47: 491 (Abstract).

27. Wang RYC, Tse TF, Yu DYC, Lee PK, Chow MSS: Haemodynamic and clinical effects of intravenous terbutaline in cardiogenic shock — a preliminary report. *Clin Pharmacol Ther* 1981; 29: 288 (Abstract).

28. Wang RYC: Management of cardiac arrhythmias. *The Hong Kong Practitioner* 1981; 3: 333–339.

29. Wang RYC: Infectious pericarditis: diagnosis and management. *Proc HK Cardiol Soc* 1981; 7: 11–16.

30. Wang RYC: Dysrhythmia quiz. *Proc HK Cardiol Soc* 1980–1981; 7: 119–127.

31. Wang RYC, Tse TF, Yu DYC, Lee PK, Chow MSS: Beneficial haemodynamic effects of terbutaline in patients with severe heart failure. *Am Heart J* 1982; 104: 1016–1021.

32. Wang RYC, Lee WT, Mok CK: Two-dimensional echocardiographic features of Bjork shiley aortic prosthetic valve dehiscence. *Thorax* 1982; 37: 540–541.

33. Woo J, Leung E, Tso N, Wang RYC: Contraception in 1980–1981 in Hong Kong. *Bull HK Med Assoc;* 34.

34. Wang RYC, Chen WC, Lee PK, Shen E: Coronary arteriographic findings among Chinese patients in Hong Kong. *Chung-Hua Nei Ko Tsa Chih* 1982; 21: 285–287.

35. Chen W, Chan CS, Lee PK, Wang R, Wang V: Pregnancy in patients with prosthetic heart valves: an experience with 45 pregnancies. *Q J Med* 1982; 51: 358–365.

36. Wong PHC, Chow JSF, Chen WWC, Wang RYC, Cheung KL, Lee JWT, Nandi PK, Mok CK: Is cardiac catheterization necessary before valvular surgery? *Med J Aust* 1982; 2Z: 363–366.

37. Wang RYC, Lee PK: The use of contrast two-dimensional echocardiography in Eisenmenger's syndrome. *Asean J Clin Sci* 1982; 3: 353–359.

38. Wang RYC, Mok CK: Erosion of an ep-

icardial pacemaker secondary to postpericardiotomy syndrome. *Pace* 1983; 6: 33–34.

39. Huang CY, Chan YW, Wang R: Senile dementia and hydrocephalus due to carotid dolicoectasia. *Clin Exp Neurol* 1983; 19: 171–176.

40. Wang RYC, Lee PK, Wong KL, Chow MSS: Mexiletine in the treatment of recurrent ventricular tachycardia — prediction of long term arrhythmia suppression from acute and short term response. *J Clin Pharmacol* 1983; 23: 89–91.

41. Kumana CR, Wang R, Chen W: Beta blocking drugs and the prophylaxis of cardiovascular disease. *The Hong Kong Practitioner* 1983; 5: 516–518.

42. Wang RYC, Cheung KL, Chen W, Lee PK, Mok CK, Ng R: Antiplatelet agents as thromboembolic prophylaxis in mechanical heart valves. *J Am Coll Cardiol* 1983; 1 (2): 700.

43. Wang RYC, Lee PK, Wong PHC: Rapid atrial fibrillation with left bundle branch block pattern in patients with Ebstein's anomaly. *Chest* 1983; 83: 814–816.

44. Chow JSF, Wang RYC, Wong PHC, Chen WWC, Lai CL: Intravenous ranitidine has no haemodynamic effects in subjects with normal lung function and patients with chronic obstructive airway disease. *Aust NZ J Med* 1983; 13: 261–263.

45. Wong CVM, Wang RYC, Tse TF: Pregnancy and Takayasu's arteritis. *Am J Med* 1983; 75: 597–601.

46. Chan KH, Chau PY, Wang RYC, Huang CY: Meningitis due to flavobacterium meningosepticum after transphenoidal hypophysectomy with recovery. *Surg Neurol* 1983; 20: 294–296.

47. Wang RYC, Lee PK, Chow JSF, Chen WWC: The use of low-dose subcutaneous heparin in pregnant women with artificial heart vales. *Med J Aust* 19083; 3: 126–128.

48. Wang RYC, Cheung KL, Lee PK, Mok CK: Diagnosis of thrombosed mitral prostheses by two dimensional echocardiography. *J Cardiovasc Ultrasonography* 1983; 2: 167–169.

49. Wang RYC, Lee PK, Yu DYC, Tse TF, Chow MSS: Myocardial metabolic effects of intravenous terbutaline in patients with severe heart failure due to coronary artery disease. *J Clin Pharmacol* 1983; 23: 362–368.

50. Wang RYC, Lee PK, Yu DYC, Tse TF, Chow MSS: Terbutaline infusion in cardiogenic shock, acute hemodynamic effects and clinical response. *J Clin Pharmacol* 1983; 23: 355–361.

51. Pan HYM, Wang RYC, Chan TK: Efficacy of two preparations of frusemide in patients with congestive heart failure. *Med J Aust*; 140: 221–222.

52. Wang RYC, Chow JSF, Chan KH, Pan HYM, Wong RPY: Acute haemodynamic and myocardial metabolic effects of intravenous urapidil in severe heart failure. *Eur Heart J* 1984; 5: 745–751.

53. Wang R: Thesis entitled 'A model for the evaluation of a new agent for the treatment of severe cardiac failure in man' was passed by the board of examiners in February 1983.

54. Lee PK, Lai CL, Lok ASF, Tse TF, Lai KN, Chow SF, Lam KC: Haemodynaemic response to intravenous cimetidine in subjects with normal lung functions and in subjects with chronic airway obstruction. *Br J Clin Pharmacol* 1981; II: 339–343.

55. Chen W, Lee PK, Chau PY: Penicillin-sensitive Moraxella prosthetic endocarditis: A near disaster due to failure to treat with penicillin. *Br Heart J* 1981; 47: 101–102.

56. Chen WC, Lee PK: Indapamide as montherapy for uncomplicated essential hypertension. *la Gazette Medicale de France*, No. 16, 1985.

57. Lee PK, Cheung KL, Lee WT, Mok CK: Pericardial effect and mediastinal mass. *Chest* 1983; 84 (4): 469–470.

58. Hui WKK, Lee PK, Chow JSF, Gibson DG: Analysis of regional left ventricular wall motion during diastole in mitral stenosis. *Br Heart J* 1983; 50: 231–239.

59. Lee PK, Cheung KL, Mok CK: Early postoperative diagnosis of free floating left atrial thrombosis by two-dimensional echocardiography. *Proc HK Cardiol Soc* 1984; 8: 137–138.

60. Wang R, Lee PK, Chow J: Experience with acute myocardial infarction in Hong Kong 1976–1982. *Proc HK Cardiol Soc* 1984; 8: 119–128.

61. Hui WKK, Cheung KL, Lee PK: Apical displacement of the anterior leaflet of the tricuspid valve. Usefulness of two-dimensional echocardiography in its differentia-

tion frosm the Ebstein's anomaly. *J Cardiovasc Ultrasonography* 1984; 3 (3): 281–283.

62. Chow JSF, Wong PC, Lee PK, Wong RYC, Chen WWC: Percutaneous transfemoral catheterisation in aortic stenosis with a USCI Sones catheter curve A type one (7540). *Cathet Cardiovasc Diagn* 1985; 11: 201–206.

63. Lee PK, Wang RYC, Chow J, Cheung KL, Wong VCC: Adjusted subcutaneous heparin in pregnant women with mechanical heart valves. *J Am Coll Cardiol* 1985; 1 (3): 392 (abstract).

64. Mok CK, Boey Js, Wang RYC, Chan TK, Cheung KL, Lee PK, Chow J, Ng RP, Tse TF: Warfarin versus clipyridamole — Aspirin and Pentoxifylline-Aspirin in the prevention of prosthetic heart valve thromboembolism: a prospective randomised clinical trial. *Circulation* 1985; 72 (5): 1059–1063.

65. Lee PK, So SY, Chow J: An unusual cause of central cyanosis in a patient with rheumatic heart disease. *Thorax* 1986; 41: 333–335.

66. Rodrigo MRC, Moles TM, Lee PK: A comparison of the incidence and nature of cardiac dysrhythmias occurring during isoflurane and halothane anaesthesia for dental surgery. *Br J Anaesth* 1985; 58: 394–400.

67. Lee PK, Wang RYC, Chow J, Cheung KL, Wong VCC, Chan TK: The combined use of warfarin and adjusted subcutaneous heparin during pregnancy in patients with artificial heart valves. *J Am Coll Cardiol* 1986; 8 (1): 221–224.

68. Mok CK, Lee PK, Boey J, Wang R, Chan TK: Preventing thromboembolism in prosthetic heart valves. *Cardiology Board Review* 1986; 3 (7): 87–95.

69. Lok ASF, Wong KP, Lee PK, Chiu KW, Mok CK, Lam SK: Radiological diagnosis of leiomyosarcoma of the inferior vena cava. *Clin Radiol* 1986; 37: 403–405.

70. Woo E, Chan FL, Yu YL, Huang CY, Chang CM, Lee PK, So SY: Bulbar palsy aggravated by metrizamide CT cisternography. *Neuroradiology* (in press).

71. Lee PK, Kerr CR, Vorderbrugge S, Qi AZ, Yeung J: Symptomatic sinus node dysfunction associated with the use of propafenone. *Am J Cardiol* (in press).

72. Chen W, Wong P, Chow J: Mitral valve prolapse and preexcitation. *Pace* 1982; 5: 773–775.

73. Chan FL, Chen W, Chow J, Wong P: Skeletal abnormalities in mitral valve prolapse. *Clin Radiol* 1983; 34: 207–213.

74. Chen W, Chan FL, Wong P, Chow J: Familial prevalence of mitral valve prolapse. is it related to straight back? *Br Heart J* 1983; 50: 97–100.

75. Wong PHC, Chow JSF, Chen WWC: Aortic catheterisation via percutaneous left ventricular puncture. *Cathet Cardiovasc Diagn* 1983; 9: 421–427.

76. Chen WC, Ng NL, Chow SF, Wong HC: Prevalence of mitral valve prolapse in Chinese. A clinical and autopsy study. *Chin Med J* 1984; 97: 352–356.

77. Pan HYM, Chow JSF: A case of haemorrhagic dengue without hypovolemia in an adult. *Trop Geogr Med* 1984; 36: 305–207.

78. Chow JSF, Wang RYC, Tang Lawrence CT, Mok CK: Right ventricular implantation of endometrial adenocarcinoma as a result of temporary pacing. *Br Med J* 1985; 290: 1249–1250.

79. Shore DF, Wong PHC, Paneth M: Results of mitral valvuloplasty with a suture plication technique. *J Thorac Cardiovasc Surg* 1980; 79: 249–257.

80. Shore DF, Wong PHC, Paneth M: The surgical management of ruptured chordae. *Circulation* 1979; 59 & 60 (Supp II): II 192.

81. Sutton M St John, Roudaut E, Dallocchio M, Wong PHC, Bricaud H, Paneth M, Gibson: Echocardiographic assessment of St. Jude mitral valve prosthesis. *Br Heart J* 1980; 43 (1): 117.

82. Wong PHC, Cotter L, Gibson D: Early systolic closure of the aortic valve. *Br Heart J* 1980; 44: 386–389.

83. Gibson D, Wong PHC: Effect of sublingual nitroglycerin on left ventricular wall movement in patients with coronary artery disease. Comparison with propanolol and saphenous bypass grafting. *La Nouvelle Press Medicale*, September 1980; 9, No. 34.

84. Wong CM, Wong PHC, Miller G: Percutaneous left ventricuar angiography. *Cathet Cardiovasc Diagn* 1981; 7: 425–432.

85. Cotter L, Wong PHC: Aortic valve closure during early or middle systole. *Herz* 1980; 5: 285–290.

86. Sutton M St John, Sutton M, Rozovsky I, Marier D, Wong PHC, Gibson D: Failure of diastolic abnormalities to regress after correction of aortic stenosis: a case for earlier correction? *Am J of Cardiol* 1980; 45: 487.

87. Wong PHC, Mok CK, Ong GB: Chylomediastinum: an unusual complication after mitral valve replacement. *Aust NZ J Surg* 1982; 52 (6): 560–561.

88. Wong PHC, Mok CK: Echocardiographic evaluation of the Hall Kaster mitral prosthesis. *Aust NZ J Surg* 1982; 52 (6): 554–558.

89. Pun KK, Wong WT, Wong PHC: The first documented outbreak of trichinellosis in Hong Kong Chinese. *Am J Trop Med Hyg* 1983; 32 (4): 772–775.

90. Wong PHC, Nandi P, Ho FCS, Chan TK: Acute severe intravascular haemolysis indicating thrombosis of Bjork-Shiley aoric prosthesis. *Arch Intern Med* 1983; 143: 1471–1472.

91. Chen WWC, Wong PHC, Chow JSF: Mitral valve prolapse and preexcitation. *Pace* 1982; 5: 773–775.

92. Wong PHC, Wong CM: The use of two dimensional echocardiography in clinical practice. *Proc HK Cardiol Soc* 1980–81; 7: 87–101.

93. Pun KK, Wong PHC: A family with fever. *The Hong Kong Practitioner*, 361–363m Bivenber 1982.

94. Wong PHC, Lee JWT: Right aortic arch and Kommerell's Diverticulum. *Thorax* 1983; 38: 553–555.

95. Nandi PL, Wong PHC, Mok CK: Corrective surgery for tetralogy of fallot in adolescents and adults. *Proceedings of the 7th Asia-Pacific Congress on Diseases of the Chest*, 82–83, Nov 1981.

96. Lau CP: Attempted suicide with enalapril. *N Engl J Med* 1986; 315: 197.

97. Wong CK, Lau CP, Leung WH: Aberrant congenital right subclavian superior vena-caval fistula in an adult cretin. *Int J Cardiol* (in press).

98. Wong CK, Lau CP, Leung WH, Cheng CH: Therapeutic trial of nifedipine in patients with Eisenmenger syndrome complicating patent ductus arteriosus. *Int J Cardiol* (in press).

99. Lau CP, Wong CK, Leung WH, Cheng CH: A comparative evaluation of minute ventilation sensing and activity sensing adaptive-rate pacemakers during daily activities. *Pacing and Clinical Electrophysiology* (in press).

100. Leung WH, Wong KL, Lau CP, Wong CK, Cheng CH, So KF: Myocardial involvement in Churg-Strauss syndrome — role of endomyocardial biopsy. *J Rheumatol* 1989; 16: 828–831.

101. Leung WH, Lau CP, Tai YT, Wong CK, Cheng CH: Candida right ventricular mural endocarditis: imaging by two-dimensional echocardiography. *Chest* (in press).

102. Leung WH, Tai YT, Lau CP, Wong CK, Cheng CH, Chan TK: Cardiac tamponade complicating acute leukemias: immediate chemotherapy versus pericardiocentesis. *Postgrad Med J* (in press).

103. Lau CP, Cheung KL, Mok CK: Biventricular perforation by a temporary pacing electrode: the role of lateral chest radiograph. *Int J Cardiol* (in press).

104. Lau CP, Leung WH, Wong CK, Cheng CH, Tai YT: Adaptive rate pacing at submaximal exercise: the importance of the programmed upper rate. *J Electrophysiol* (in press).

105. Leung WH, Pun KK, Lau CP, Wong CK, Wang C: Amiodarone-induced thyroiditis. *Am Heart J* (in press).

106. Lau CP, Leung WH, Wong CK, Cheng CH, Tai YT: Adaptive rate pacing at submaximal exercise: the importance of a critically programmed upper rate. *J Electrophysiol* (in press).

107. Lau CP, Leung WH, Wong CK, Cheng CH: Haemodynamics of induced atrial fibrillation: a comparative assessment with sinus rhythm, atrial and ventricular pacing. *Eur Heart J* (in press).

108. Leung WH, Lau CP, Wong CK, Leung CY: Fatal cardiac tamponade in systemic lupus erythematosis — a hazard of anticoagulation. *Am heart J* (in press).

109. Wong CK, Leung WH, Cheng CH, Lau CP: Myxomatous mitral valve degeneration complicating asymptomatic cor triatriatum. *Clin Cardiol* 1989; 12: 48–50.

110. Wong CK, Cheng CH, Lau CP, Leung WH, Chan FL: Interrupted aortic arch in an asymptomatic adult. *Chest* 1988 (in press).

111. Lau CP, Wong CK, Leung WH, Cheng CH: Ultrasonic assisted permanent pacing in a patient with destroyed lung complicating pulmonary tuberculosis. *Pacing and Clinical Electrophysiology* 1989 (in press).

112. Leung WH, Wong CK, Lau CP, Cheng CH: Cor triatriatum in an dult masked by coexisting chronic obstructive pulmonary disease in adulthood. *Chest* 1988 (in press).

113. Wong CK, Lau CP, Cheng CH, Leung WH, Chan TYK, Pun KK: Elevated atrial naturetic factor in giant right atrium complicating Marfan's syndrome. *Eur Heart J* 1988 (in press).

114. Leung WH, Lau CP, Wong CK, Cheng CH, Tai YT: Improvement in exercise performance and hemodynamics by labetalol in idiopathic dilated cardiomyopathy. *Am Heart J* (in press).

115. Wong CK, Cheng CH, Lau CP, Leung WH: Congenital coronary artery anomalies in Noonan's syndrome. *Am Heart J* (in press).

116. Leung WH, Lau CP, Wong CK: Left ventricular mural endocarditis. *Am Heart J* (in press).

117. Wong CK, Cheng CH, Lau CP, Leung WH: Asymptomatic congenital coronary artery aneurysm in adulthood. *Eur Heart J* (in press).

118. Lau CP: Pacemakers that give more energy. *Journal of Hong Kong General Practitioner* 1989, January issue.

119. Lau CP, Leung WH, Wong CK, Cheng CH, So SY: Electrical ablation of the atrioventricular node for the control of junctional tachycardia in a patient with amiodarone induced pulmonary fibrosis. *J HK Med Assoc* (in press).

120. Leung WH, Lau CP, Cheng CH, Wong CK, Tai YT: Beta adrenoceptor blockade in congestive cardiac failure. *J HK Med Assoc* (submitted for publication).

121. Chen WWC, Tai YT: Dissection of interventricular system by aneurysm of sinus of Valsalva: a rare complication diagnosed by echocardiography. *Br Heart J* 1983; 50: 293–295.

122. Wong KL, Tai YT, Lok SL, Woo EKW, Wong WS, Chan MK, Ma JTC: Disseminated zygomycosis masquerading as cerebral lupus erythematosus. *Am J Clin Pathol* 1986; 86: 546–549.

123. Wong RWS, Wong MB, Tai YT: Penicillamine-induced polymyositis in rheumatoid arthritis. *Asean J Clin Sci* 1988; 8: 85–87.

124. Yusoff K, Tai YT, Campbell RWF: Hemodynamic consequences of supraventricular tachycardias and their antiarrhythmic treatment. *Zweiscript de Kardiologie* 1989 (in press).

125. Tai YT, Campbell RWF, McComb JM: Latent functional duality in an accessary pathway. *Eur Heart J* 1989; 10: 380–384.

126. Tai YT, Lo CW, Chow WH, Cheng CH: Successful resuscitation and survival following massive overdose of metoprolol. *Br J Clin Practice* (in press).

127. Tai YT, Mok CK, Chow WH: Left ventricular pseudoaneurysm after replacement of the mitral valve: long term survival and spontaneous closure. *Int J Cardiol* 1989 (in press).

128. Chow WH, Tai YT, Cheung KL: False detection of left atrial thrombus by the angiographic sign of 'neovascularity'. *Cathet Cardiovasc Diagn* 1989 (in press).

129. Chow WH, Cheng CH, Chow L, Cheung KL, Tai YT: Percutaneous balloon mitral valvoplasty. *J HK Med Assoc* 1989 (in press).

130. Chow WH, Cheng CH, Tse TM, Cheung KL: Tracheal stenosis after endotracheal intubation and assisted ventilation. *J HK Med Assoc* 1988; 40 (2).

131. Lau CP, Cheng CH, Leung WH, Wong CK: The use of cardiac electrophysiology study in the management of patients with cardiac arrhythmias. *HK Cardiol Soc* 1988 Biennial Scientific Congress 19–20th November 1988 (abstract).

132. Cheng CH, Cheung KL, Chow WH, Lau CP, Mok CK, Cheung D, Lee J: Coronary artery disease in the elderly Chinese — Experience at the Grantham Hospital. *HK Cardiol Soc, 1988 Biennial Scientific Congress, 19–20th November 1988* (Abstract).

133. Chow WH, Cheng CH, Cheung KL: Incidence of coronary artery disease in patients with valvular heart disease in Hong Kong. *HK Cardiol Soc 1988 Biennial Scientific Congress, 19–20th November 1988* (Abstract).

134. Lau CP, Cheng CH, Wu WZ, Lee PK, Chow JSF, Wang RYC: Risk factors and natural history of acute myocardial infarction in Hong Kong. *HK Cardiol Soc, 1988 Biennial*

Scientific Congress, 19–20th November 1988 (Abstract).

135. Cheung DLC, Mok CK, Lee WT, Cheung KL, Cheng CH, Chow WH, Chow L: Coronary artery bypass surgery for unstable angina pectoris. *HK Cardiol Soc, 1988 Biennial Scientific Congress, 19–20th November 1988* (Abstract).

136. Lau CP, Wong CK, Cheng CH, Leung WH: Comparative assessment of the rate responses of a minute ventilation sensing and an activity sensing rate modulated pacemaker to normal daily activities. *HK Cardiol Soc, 1988 Biennial Scientific Congress, 19–20th November 1988* (Abstract).

137. Lee WT, Mok CK, Cheung D, Cheung KL, Cheng CH: Aortic valve replacement in patients with grossly dilated left ventricle. *HK Cardiol Soc, 1988 Biennial Scientific Congress, 19–20th November 1988* (Abstract).

138. Wong CK, Lau CP, Leung WH, Cheng CH: Therapeutic trial of Nifedipine in patients with Eisenmenger syndrome complicating patent ductus arteriosus. *1st International Symposium on Heart Failure-mechanisms and Management, Jerusalem, Israel May 1989* (Abstract).

139. Leung WH, Lau CP, Cheng CH, Wong CK, Tai YT, Lo CW: Beneficial effect of combined alpha and beta blockade of labetalol in idiopathic dilated cardiomyopaty. *1st International Symposium on Heart Failure-mechanisms and Management, Jerusalem, Israel May 1988* (Abstract).

140. Lau CP, Leung WH, Tai YT, Wong CK, Cheng CH, Tam C: Regularization and rate control of atrial fibrillation using intercalated ventricular pacing. *10th Annual Scientific Session, North American Society of Pacing and Electrophysiology May 1989* (Abstract).

141. Lau CP, Cheng CH, Muro C, Tse M, Tai YT, Leung WH, Wong CK, Cheung KL, Chow WH, Wu PC: Attitudes towards cardiac pacing amongst doctors in Hong Kong. *4th Asian-Pacific Symposium on Cardiac Pacing and electrophysiology, August, Singapore;* p. 13 (Abstract).

142. Lau CP, Leung WH, Wong CK, Tai YT, Cheng CH, Tam C: A new pacing method for regularization and rate control of atrial fibrillation. *4th Asian-Pacific Symposium on Cardiac Pacing and Electrophysiology, August, Singapore,* p. 163 (Abstract).

143. Lau CP, Leung WH, Wong CK, Cheng CH, Tai YT: Adaptive-rate pacing during submaximal exercise — the importance of a critically programmed upper rate. *4th Asian-Pacific Symposium on Cardiac Pacing and Electrophysiology, August, Singapore,* p. 191 (Abstract).

144. Lau CP, Wong CK, Leung WH, Cheng CH, Lo CW: An evaluation of minute ventilation sensing and activity sensing adaptive-rate pacemakers during daily activities. *4th Asian-Pacific Symposium on Cardiac Pacing and Electrophysiology, August, Singapore,* p. 192 (Abstract).

145. Lau CP, Leung WH, Wong CK, Cheng CH: Haemodynamics of induced atrial fibrillation. *4th Asian-Pacific Symposium on Cardiac Pacing and Electrophysiology, August, Singapore,* p. 214 (Abstract).

146. Yan V, Hunt D, Sloman G: Pericardial pain in acute myocardial infarction, double blind trial of steroid therapy. *Eur J Cardiol* 1973; 1: 79.

**Chun Ho CHENG,
Y.T. TAI and C.P. LAU**

Division of Cardiology in Grantham Hospital

The Grantham Hospital was opened in 1957 as a tuberculosis hospital under the operation of the Hong Kong Tuberculosis, Chest and Heart Disease Association (The Association). An open heart unit, the first in Hong Kong, was started at the Grantham Hospital in 1968 and in 1974 a working party consisting of Prof. D. Todd and others was set up by the Association to develop Grantham Hospital into a major cardiothoracic centre for the prevention, treatment and rehabilitation of patients with heart diseases. This proposal was supported by government and the project became a joint venture of the Association and the Hong Kong Heart Foundation Ltd. With such joint efforts and the generous donation by Mr. Kwok Tak Sing, a cardiac catheterization laboratory was set up in 1979, a 2-dimensional echocardiographic (2D echo) machine in 1982 and a fully functioning cardiac centre, the Kwok Tak Sing Heart Centre, was opened on 11 March 1982 at the Grantham Hospital. A cardiac medical unit, headed by Prof. David Todd, was also established.

Clinical Services

The Cardiac Unit continues to expand and modernize after its establishment: — a cardiac OPD was started in 1982 and a CCU with 8 beds was opened in 1983. With the rapid advances in cardiac technology and increasing demand for cardiac investigations and treatment, recurrent requests were made for more modern equipments and upgrading of old ones and the unit now has 2 holter analyzers with 12 recorders, 1 treadmill machine, 4 respirators, 1 telemetry with 4 channels, 1 intra-aortic balloon counter-pulsation machine, 2 2D echo doppler machine and a new colour-coded 2D echo doppler machine of the latest model under tender. A new cardiac catheterization machine with modern cardiac digital imaging has been requested repeatedly over the past 4 to 5 years but was still not granted probably because of its high cost (> 15 million). The purchase of expensive modern equipments is however well justified considering the tremendous and ever expanding service in cardiology

offered at the Grantham Hospital as reflected by the following statistics of the Adult Cardiac Medical Unit alone: —

Number of:	1982	1988
Cardiac Catheterization	297	594
24 Hour holter monitoring	—	465
Exercise treadmill test	—	259
2D echo (doppler) study	2,000	>12,000
OPD out-patients	2,030	19,982

The number of out-patients clinics have increased from three, 1 general cardiac and 2 valvular (anticoagulation), to seven with the addition of 2 echo clinics, 1 pacemaker clinic and 1 PTCA clinic. The cardiac unit in Grantham Hospital has not just expanded but has also been keeping pace with the rapid advances in new therapy and technology for cardiac diseases. It has pioneered in the field of interventional cardiology in Hong Kong such as percutaneous transluminal coronary angioplasty (PTCA), percutaneous balloon valvuloplasty (56, 57) and embolization of arterial-venous malformation and percutaneous trans-arterial and venous retrieval of foreign bodies (33). The first successful PTCA was performed at the Grantham Hospital in December 1984, the first pulmonary valvuloplasty in April 1986, the first mitral valvuloplasty in June 1988 and the first tricuspid valvuloplasty on a bioprosthesis in February 1989 (59).

Research

Despite the heavy clinical workload in cardiology at the Grantham Hospital, research is not forgotten. As the Grantham cardiac medical and surgical units work closely together with good cooperation, majority of the research studies were the combined efforts of the 2 teams. Early studies include prevention of cardiac tamponade after open heart surgery (1, 3), methods of treatment of various congenital heart diseases (2, 5, 9, 13), reviews of surgical treatment of various congenital heart diseases (4, 8, 11), and post-operative studies on patients after valvular surgery (6,

7, 39, 40, 60). Unusual complications of open heart surgery such as malaria and chylomediastinum, specific complications of mitral valve replacement such as floating LA thrombus (26) and outlet strut fracture of the Bjork Shiley convexoconcave mitral valve prosthesis (32). Unusual complications of cardiac pacing such as erosion of epicardial pacemaker secondary to postpericardiotomy syndrome (21), right ventricular implantation of endometrial adenocarcinoma and biventricular perforation after temporary pacing (29), (45) were reported. The extensive studies on thromboembolic prophylaxis in mechanical heart valves (18, 23, 25, 31, 33, 34, 35), and in particular the prospective randomized clinical trial on Warfarin versus dipyridamole-aspirin and pentoxifylline-aspirin for the prevention of prosthetic heart valve thromboembolism (33) has received international recognition and the studies on subcutaneous heparin in pregnant women with mechanical heart valves (18, 23, 31) have aroused interest of not only cardiologists but also obstetricians all over the world. Various papers were published on the use of 2D echo-doppler as a diagnostic tool on valvular heart diseases (16) aortic prosthetic valve dehiscence (14) coronary AV fistula (20, 30) acquired aortic-RV fistula (51), thrombosed mitral prosthesis (22), floating LA thrombus (26, 53) and in differentiating apical displacement of anterior leaflet of the tricuspid valve from true Ebstein's anamoly (28). Interesting and unusual radiological features of pericardial effusion (24), the thoracic arota (38) and LA thrombus (54) were reported. In recent years, with the increasing awareness of coronary artery disease in Hong Kong, increasing number of patients are subjected to coronary angiography, aorto-coronary bypass graft surgery (CABG) and PTCA. Our local experience and studies on these patients with coronary artery disease were published (41, 42, 43, 47, 50, 52). The diagnosis and treatment of acute dissecting aneurysm of the aorta (27) and rare but interesting clinical presentations of cardiac diseases were also reported (36, 37, 49, 55, 57).

Teaching

Besides clinical service and research, the Grantham Hospital has also served as a teaching hospital in cardiology for both undergraduates and post-graduates. Renowned cardiologists from overseas were impressed after their visits to the hospital. It has built up its reputation over the years and medical students as well as post-graduate doctors were sent here for their training in cardiology not just from Hong Kong but also from the United Kingdom, the United States, Australia and China.

Acknowledgement

The achievement in cardiology in Grantham Hospital over the past 15 years as described above were made possible by the combined efforts and support of the University Department Heads, the Medical & Health Department, the Hong Kong Tuberculosis, Chest and Heart Disease Association, the H.K. Heart Foundation and all those who have worked here. The cardiologists serving in the hospital since 1974 are: Dr. K.L. Cheung (10/74 to date), Dr. Philip H.C. Wong (1/80–11/81), Dr. Walter W.C. Chen (9/82–12/83), Dr. P.K. Lee (9/82–4/83, 6/85–6/87), Dr. William K.K. Hui (9/83–6/84), Dr. Rebecca Y.C. Wang (1/84–5/85), Dr. C.H. Cheng (Part-time 7/85–7/87), Dr. W.H. Chow (12/87 to date), Dr. Simon L. Chow (2/88–10/88), Dr. Y.T. Tai (Part-time 1/89–6/89) and Dr. T.M. Tse (7/89 to date).

Publications

1. Nandi P, Cheung KL, Leung JSM: Closure of pericardium after open heart surgery. A way to prevent post-operative cardiac tamponade. *British Heart Journal* 1976; 38: 1319–1323.
2. Nandi P, Mok CK, Cheung KL, Ong GB: Surgery of isolated patent ductus arteriosus — Review of 188 cases. *Southeast Asian Journal of Surgery* 1978; 1(1): 43–50.
3. Nandi P, Mok CK, Cheung KL, Ong GB: Open-heart surgery and post-operative cardiac tamponade. *Southeast Asian Journal of Surgery* 1978; 1(1): 62–69.
4. Nandi P, Mok CK, Cheung KL, Ong GB: Ventricular septal defect associated with aortic regurgitation — Review of 11 surgically treated cases. *Malaysian Journal of Surgery* 1978; 4: 63–65.

5. Mok CK, Cheung KL, Kong SM, Ong GB: Translocating the aberrant right subclavian artery in dysphagia lusoria. *British Journal of Surgery* 1979; 66: 113–116.

6. Nandi P, Mok CK, Cheung KL, Ong GB: Surgery for aortic valve disease in Hong Kong — 10-year Chinese experience. *Philippine Journal of Cardiology* 1979; 7: 139–145.

7. Lee WT, Mok CK, Cheung KL, Ong GB: Mitral valve replacement in children and adolescents. *Proceedings of the Hong Kong Cardiological Society* 1979; 6: 145–160.

8. Nandi P, Mok CK, Cheung KL, Lee WT, Ong GB: Coarctation of the aorta — Review of surgical experience in Hong Kong. *Singapore Medical Journal* 1979; 20: 430–433.

9. Mok CK, Chan MC, Cheung KL, Lee WT, Nandi P, Ong GB: Early intracardiac repair of large ventricular septal defect with conventional cardiopulmonary bypass and moderate hypothermia. *Australian & New Zealand Journal of Surgery* 1980; 50: 378–381.

10. Mok CK, Cheung KL, Wei KH, Ong GB: Malaria complicating open-heart surgery. *Thorax* 1980; 35: 389–391.

11. Nandi P, Mok CK, Cheung KL, Lee WT, Ong GB: Total correction of tetralogy of Fallot. *Journal of Royal College of Surgeons of Edinburgh* 1981; 26: 340–343.

12. CM Wong, PHC Wong, GAH Miller: Percutaneous left ventricular angiography. *Catheterization and Cardiovascular Diagnosis* 1981; 7: 425–432.

13. Mok CK, Lee WT, Nandi P, Cheung KL, Ong GB: Early correction of cardiac anomalies using extracorporeal circulation. *Journal of Royal College of Surgeons of Edinburgh* 1982; 27: 33–37.

14. Wang R, Lee WT, Mok CK; Two-dimensional echocardiographic features of Bjork Shiley aortic prosthetic valve dehiscence. *Thorax* 1982; 37: 540–541.

15. Chen W, Mok CK, Ng WL: Haemoptysis in pulmonary artery aneurysm associated with pulmonary hypertension: Surgical dilemma. *Australian & New Zealand Journal of Surgery* 1982; 52: 557–559.

16. Wong PHC, Chow JSF, Chen WWC, Wang RYC, Cheung KL, Lee JWT, Nandi P, Mok CK: Is cardiac catheterization necessary before valvular surgery? *Medical Journal of Australia* 1982; 2: 363–366.

17. Wong PHC, Mok CK: Echocardiographic assessment of the Hall-Kaster mitral prosthesis. *Australian & New Zealand Journal of Surgery* 1982; 52: 554–557.

18. Chen W, Chan CS, Lee PK, Wang R, Wang V: Pregnancy in patients with prosthetic heart valves: an experience with 45 pregnancies. *Quartrly Journal of Medicine* 1982; 51: 358–365.

19. Wong PHC, Mok CK, Ong GB: Chylomediastinum: An unusual complication after mitral valve replacement. *Australian & New Zealand Journal of Surgery* 1982; 52: 560–561.

20. Chen W, Woo KS, Kong SM and Mok CK: Coronary artery to left ventricle fistulas: echocardiographic features. *Cardiovasc Intervent Radiol* 1982; 5: 241–245.

21. Wang RYC, Mok CK: Erosion of an epicardial pacemaker secondary to postpericardiotomy syndrome. *Pace* 1983; 6: 33–34.

22. Wang RYC, Cheung KL, Lee PK, Mok CK: Diagnosis of thrombosed mitral prosthesis by two-dimensional echocardiography. *Journal of Cardiovascular Ultrasonography* 1983; 2: 167–169.

23. Wang RYC, Lee PK, Chow JSF, Chen WWC: The use of low-dose subcutaneous heparin in pregnant women with artifical heart valves. *The Medical Journal of Australia* 1983; 3: 126–128.

24. Lee PK, Lee JWT, Cheung KL, Mok CK: Pericardial effusion and mediastinal mass. *Chest* 1983; 84: 469–470.

25. Wang RYC, Cheung KL, Chen WWC, Lee PK, Mok CK, Ng RP: Antiplatelet agents as thromboembolic prophylaxis in mechanical valves. *Journal of American College of Cardiology* 1983; 1(2): 700.

26. Lee PK, Cheung KL, Mok CK: Early postoperative diagnosis of free floating left atrial thrombus by two-dimensional echocardiography. *Proceedings of the Hong Kong Cardiological Society* 1984; 8: 137–138.

27. Wang R, Lee PK, Chow J, Cheung KL, Lee WT, Mok CK: Acute dissecting aneurysm of the aorta: diagnosis and treatment. *Proceedings of the Hong Kong Cardiological Soceity* 1984; 8: 105–110.

28. Hui WKK, Cheung KL, Lee PK: Apical displacement of the anterior leaflet of the tricuspid valve: Usefulness of two-dimensional echocrdiography in its differentia-

tion from true Ebstein's anamoly. *Journal of Cardiovascular Ultrasonography* 1984; 3: 281–283.

29. Chow JSF, Wang RYC, Tang LCH, Mok CK: Right ventricular implantation of endometrial adenocarcinoma as as result of temporary pacing. *British Medical Journal* 1985; 290: 1249–1250.

30. Mok CK, Cheung KL, Wang RYC: An unruptured right-coronary sinus to left ventricle aneurysm diagnosed by two-dimensional echocardiography. *British Heart Journal* 1985; 53: 226–229.

31. Lee PK, Wang RYC, Chow JSF, Cheung KL, Wong VCW: Adjusted subcutaneous heparin in pregnant women with mechanical heart valve. Journal of American College of Cardiology 1985; 1(3): 392(Abstract).

32. Mok CK, Lee JWT, Kong SM, Hui KK: Experience with outlet strut fracture of the Bjork Shiley convexoconcave mitral valve prosthesis. *American Heart Journal* 1985; 110: 814–818.

33. Mok CK, Boey J, Wang RYC, Chan TK, Cheung KL, Lee PK, Chow J, Ng RP, Tse TF: Warfarin versus dipyridamole-aspirin and pentoxifylline-aspirin for the prevention of prosthetic heart valve thromboembolism: A prospective randomized clinical trail. *Circulation* 1985; 72(5): 1059–1063.

34. Mok CK, Lee PK, Boey J, Wang R, Chan TK: Preventing thrombolism in prosthetic heart valves. *Cardiology Board Review* 1986; 3: 87–95.

35. Lee PK, Wang RYC, Chow J, Cheung KL, Wong VCC: The combined use of warfarin and adjusted subcutaneous heparin during pregnancy in patients with artifical heart valves. *Journal of American College of Cardiology* 1986; 8(1): 221–224.

36. Chow WH, Cheung KL: Primary hepatocellular carcinoma masquerading as infective endocarditis. *British Medical Journal* 1986; 292. 1364

37. Lee Jan, Cheung KL, Wang R, Mok CKB, Khin MA: Malignant fibrous histiocytoma of left atrium. *The Journal of Thoracic and Cardiovascular Surgery* Sept. 1987; 94 (3): 450–452.

38. Mok CK, Cheung KL, Chan FL, Leung MP: Left aortic arch with right descending aorta. *Australian Radiology* Aug. 1988; 32 (3).

39. Lee WT, Mok CK, Cheung D, Cheung KL, Cheng CH: Aortic valve replacement in patients with grossly dilated left ventricle. *Proceedings of 1988 Biennial Scientific Congress.*

40. Cheung DLC, Mok CK, Lee WT, Cheung KL: Surgical treatment of active bacterial endocarditis — an analysis of ten year experience in Hong Kong. *Proceedings of 1988 Biennial Scientific Congress.*

41. Cheng CH, Cheung KL, Chow WH, Lau CP, Mok CK, Cheung D, Lee J: Coronary artery disease in the elderly Chinese — Experience at the Grantham Hospital. *Proceedings of 1988 Biennial Scientific Congress.*

42. Chow WH, Cheng CH, Cheung KL: Incidence of coronary artery disease in pateints with valvular heart disease in Hong Kong. *Proceedings of 1988 Biennial Scientific Congress.*

43. Cheung DLC, Mok CK, Lee WT, Cheung KL, Cheng CH, Chow WH, Chow L: Coronary artery bypass surgery for unstable angina pectoris. *Proceedings of 1988 Biennial Scientific Congress.*

44. Chow WH, Cheng CH, Tse TM, Cheung KL: Tracheal stenosis after endotracheal intubation and assisted ventilation. *Journal of the Hong Kong Medical Association* 1988; 40(2): 143–144.

45. Lau CP, Cheung KL and Mok CK: Biventricular perforation by a temporary pacing electrode: recognition from the lateral chest radiography. *International Journal of Cardiology* 1989.

46. Chow WH, Cheung KL, Ling HM, See T: Potentiation of warfarin anticoagulation by topical methylsalicylate ointment. *Journal of the Royal Society of Medicine* 1989; 82: 501–502.

47. Chow WH, Cheung KL, Cheng CH: Total occlusion of the left main coronary artery in a Hong Kong Chinese. *Chinese Medical Journal* 1989; 102: 227–229.

48. Chow WH, Chow L, Cheung KL, Lee J, Khin A: Infected atrial myxoma. *Postgraduate Medical Journal* 1989; 65: 671–673.

49. Chow WH: Survival of a patient with an infected right atrial myxoma following surgery (Letter). *Eurpoean Heart Journal* 1989; 10: 87.

50. Chow WH: Iatrogenic left main coronary

artery stenosis following aortic valve replacement (Letter). *Eurpoean Heart Journal* 1989; 10: 482.

51. Chow WH, Lee PK, Cheung KL, Mok CK: Two-dimensional and pulsed Doppler echocardiographic diagnosis of an acquired aortic-right ventricular fistula. *Clinical Cardiology* 1989; 12: 544–545.

52. Fishell T, Tse TM, Stadus M: Coronary artery spasm routinely occurs after PTCA. *Circulation* February 1989.

53. Chow WH, Chow L, Cheung KL, Lee WT: Free floating left atrial ball thrombus in a Hong Kong Chinese. *Proceedings of PUMC and CAS* (in press).

54. Chow WH, Tai YT, Cheung KL: False detection of left atrial thrombus by the angiographic sign of 'neovascularity'. Catheterization and Cardiovascular Diagnosis 1989 (in press).

55. Chow WH, Cheung KL, Lee TCB: Enhancement of warfarin anticoagulation in thyrotoxicosis. *International Journal of Clinical Practice* (in press).

56. Chow WH, Cheng CH, Chow L, Cheung KL, Tai YT: Percutaneous mitral balloon valvuloplasty. *Journal of the Hong Kong Medical Association 1989* (in press).

57. Chow WH, Cheung KL: Pulsatile varicose veins — a sign of tricuspid regurgitation. *British Journal of Clinical Practice* 1989 (in press).

58. Tai TY, Mok CK, Chow WH: Left ventricular pseudoaneurysm following surgical repair of ventricular rupture post-mitral valvular replacement: long term survival and spontaneous closure. *International Journal of Cardiology* (in press).

59. Chow WH, Cheung KL, Tai YT, Cheng CH: Successful percutaneous balloon dilatation of a stenotic tricuspid bioprosthesis. *American Heart Journal* (in press).

60. Lee WT, Mok CK, Cheung LC, Chow WH, Cheung KL: Reconstructive surgery on the mitral valve (accepted for presentation on the 9th Biennial Asian Congress on Thoracic and Cardiovascular Surgery).

K.L. CHEUNG

ACHIEVEMENTS IN CLINICAL PHARMACOLOGY

Clinical Pharmacology, a discipline complementary to yet distinct from basic pharmacology, was introduced into the medical faculty of HKU in 1982 and currently forms part of the Department of Medicine. Its continuing achievements and long-term overall objectives include the following:

Heightening awareness of Clinical Pharmacology and the importance of what it can offer clinicians: First and foremost, this is because treatment with drugs is frequently the final common pathway of medical practice, and deserves at least as much forethought, effort and attention as do diagnostic (clinical and investigative) skills. Secondly, technological advances have generally made the diagnostic aspects of clinical medicine easier, whilst modern therapeutics has become much more complex due to the wealth of ever increasing knowledge and confusion about whether or not and how individual drugs should be used. Thirdly, today's prescriber is also confronted with a vast array of similar (me too) drugs belonging to any given class, and it therefore becomes essential to develop a sensible, practical and scientific approach towards coping with the various claims and counter claims about their respective benefits and adverse effects.

Continuous refinement, review and updating of educational activity, whilst establishing only a relatively limited number of formal lectures: Being aware of the pressure on medical students and the information explosion they are faced with, there has been a deliberate attempt to: (a) reduce the emphasis on the assimilation of unnecessary factual details whilst promoting greater awareness of principles and (b) advocate the application of such principles to individual issues (and cases) by encouraging students to seek out and refer to appropriate resources.

The efficient and harmonious development of Clinical Pharmacology within the Faculty of Medicine: The need for utmost cooperation with Clinical departments (especially individual clinicians within the Department of Medicine), the Department of Pharmacology and the Clinical Chemistry Unit has been fully recognized and actively nurtured. In order to promote close links with other disciplines, establishment of joint research projects, educational activities and other contacts have been established and must continue to grow. By these means, Clinical Pharmacology can confidently win the respect and appreciation of other specialties, become fully integrated in the work of the faculty and make a significant contribution to its achievements.

Educational Activities

A comprehensive educational framework in Clinical Pharmacology and Therapeutics for both medical students and staff has been organized. There has also been input into Clinical Pharmacology teaching for dental students as well as those studying for various other degrees and diplomas (Certificate of Medical Science, Extra mural studies in Pharmacology). Ensuing from such efforts perhaps, an awareness of Clinical Pharmacology and its importance to the scientific practice of therapeutics has begun to emerge, where previously there had been very little insight. Although this trend is evident both within the Faculty of Medicine and amongst practitioners in the community, much greater awareness needs to be fostered. The most important contributions/commitments to Clinical Pharmacology education can be summarized as follows:

1. A course of lectures in Clinical Pharmacology and Therapeutics (held annually) organized for 4th year M.B. students.
2. Conduct of a series of small group seminars/tutorials in Clinical Pharmacology, for final year M.B. students (during each clinical clerkship in medicine).
3. Organization and presentation of regular Therapeutic Conferences attended by junior and senior staff in the Department of Medicine (and other departments), final year M.B. students, and by other doctors practicing within and outside Queen Mary Hospital.
4. Organization/supervision of an experiment in Clinical Pharmacology (Pharmacology Practical course for 2nd year M.B. students).
5. Book reviews and forwards as well as educational articles in local journals — on im-

portant aspects of Clinical Pharmacology and Therapeutics (see list of publications).

6. Lecturing by invitation on various aspects of Clinical Pharmacology — to a variety of different organizations, viz. General Practitioners, Dental Practitioners, Clinical Chemists, Pharmacists, Pharmaceutical representatives, Medical Colleges in the Republic of China.

7. Moderation/Chairmanship at various seminars, conferences and refresher courses for Specialists and General Practitioners.

8. Involvement on behalf of local academic societies, viz. (i) The Hong Kong Pharmacology Society (Founding Member and former Secretary), (ii) The Hong Kong Society of Antimicrobial Chemotherapy (Founder member and current President).

9. Provision of in-depth and detailed drug information. This has been achieved through books, journals and access to other resources. The Iowa Drug Information System (IDIS) microfiche service, was introduced as a tool of Clinical Pharmacology for the faculty library. More recently the Department of Medicine has acquired direct computerized access to international drug data bases.

Special Interests and Research Projects

Clinical Pharmacology in its broadest sense, is the scientific study of therapeutic and non-therapeutic drug use (and abuse) in humans. Special attention and effort has been directed towards aspects deemed to be particularly relevant or unique to the local population. Such aspects include: inter-ethnic differences in drug dose response relationships, difficulties and unique features of drug prescribing, drug dispensing and drug delivery to local patients, and the extent of patient co-operation and understanding about the medicines they take. Accordingly, the following special interests/research projects have evolved:

1. *Search for clinically significant peculiarities of drug usage/prescribing in Hong Kong, viz.:*
   a) Discovery of very widespread community use of chloramphenicol but no apparent link with aplastic anaemia
   b) A high prevalence of dental discolouration has been linked to excessive exposure of local children to tetracyclines (liquid formulations). Since publicizing our data such exposure has fallen.
   c) Hospital and non-hospital sales of parenteral and oral cephalosporins and parenteral and topical aminoglycosides were found to be distinctly different from corresponding sales in western countries.
   d) Anti-asthmatic drug utilization (quantitative and qualitative aspects) — has been reviewed in relation to local asthma mortality.

2. *Search for possible clinically relevant inter-ethnic pharmacokinetic differences:*
   a) Distribution differences of fat soluble drugs has been found in the relatively lean Chinese.
   b) Acetylator phenotypes in H.K. SLE patients and controls have been determined.

3. *Provision of drug information to patients — by supplying information sheets and evaluation of their educational impact,* has been shown to be of limited benefit.

4. *Exposure to hepatotoxic pyrrolizidine alkaloids through the prevailing popularity of traditional folk (herbal) medicines in the community,* has been thoroughly investigated following a small outbreak of such poisoning.

5. *Involvement with drug regulatory authorities concerning drugs widely regarded as having unacceptable adverse effects* (e.g. dipyrone), and the steps being taken to control their use or deregister them.

6. *Active participation in the design, organization and conduct of randomized clinical drug trials pertinent to Hong Kong, viz.:*
   a) Therapeutic and prophylactic studies involving antimicrobials.
   b) IV glycerol for acute strokes.
   c) Drug absorption in diabetic patients taking Guar Gum dietary fibre.

7. *Involvement with drug administration and dispensing procedures:* This entailed introduction of a totally new Drug Order Form, which includes a system for recording drug orders executed by nurses — now used in all wards of the Department of Medicine at Queen Mary Hospital. The adoption of universal, computerized Drug labelling and possibly also a coding system for identifying tablets and capsules is also being advocated.

8. *Evaluation (in local patients) of bioavailability differences between brand name medicines and generic substitutes used in Hong Kong.*

Scientific Publications 1983–1989 (including Reviews and Chapters in Books but excluding Abstracts)

1. Kumana CR, Ng M, Lin HJ, Ko W, Wu DC, Todd D: Hepatic veno-occlusive disease due to toxic alkaloid exposure in herbal tea. *Lancet* 1983; 2: 1360–1361.
   N.B. The above report prompted a Lancet Editorial entitled Phrrolizidine Alkaloids (*Lancet* 1984, 1, 201–202.)
2. Kumana CR, Ogle CW: A class experiment in clinical pharmacology using beta adrenoceptor antagonist drugs. *Br J Clin Pharm* 1985; 19: 169–175.
3. Kumana CR, Ng M, Lin HJ, Ko W, Wu DC, Todd D: Herbal tea induced hepatic veno-occlusive disease: quantification of toxic alkaloid exposure in adults. *Gut* 1985; 26: 101–104.
4. Kumana CR, Tanser PH, Eydt J: Life threatening ventricular arrhythmias provoked by amiodarone. *Hum Toxicol* 1985; 4: 169–176.
5. Kumana CR, Chau KK, Chau PY, Kou M, Lauder I: Chemoprophylaxis with oral amoxycillin against bacterial endocarditis; when should second doses be administered after dentistry? *Br Med J* 1986; 293: 1532–1534.
6. Kumana CR: The role of selective beta adrenoceptor antagonists in the treatment of hypertension. In: *Proceedings of a Symposium on 'Prevention in Cardiovascular Disease — New Concepts and Developments'* (ed. Mahon WA), Ciba Geigy, Canada Ltd., 1986, pp. 71–77.
7. Culvenor CCJ, Edgar JA, Smith LW, Kumana CR, Lin HJ: Heliotropium lasiocarpum fisch and mey identified as cause of veno-occlusive disease due to a herbal tea. *Lancet* 1986; 1: 978.
8. Kumana CR: Beta adrenergic blocking drugs. *Drugs for Heart Disease*, 2nd edition (ed. Hamer J), Chapman & Hall Ltd., London, England, 1987; Ch 2, pp. 29–75.
9. Zhao X, Chan MY, Kumana CR, Ogle CW: A comparative study on the pyrrolizidine alkaloid content and the pattern of hepatic pyrrolic metabolite accumulation in mice given extracts of eupatorium plant species, crotalaria assamica and an Indian herbal mixture. *Am J Chin Med* 1987; 15: 59–67.
10. Kumana CR, Lauder IJ, Chan M, Ko W, Lin HJ: Differences in diazepam pharmacokinetics in Chinese and white Caucasians: relation to body lipid stores. *Euro J Clin Pharmacol* 1987; 32: 211–215.
11. Kumana CR: Are blood pressure surges associated with sympathetic stimulation aggravated by beta-adrenoceptor antagonist treatment? *Postgrad Med J* 1986; 62: 731–735.
12. Kumana CR, Li KY, Chau PY: Worldwide variation in use of chloramphenicol. *Lancet* 1987; 2: 449–450.
13. Kumana CR: Analgesics, agranulocytosis and aplastic anaemia. *J Am Med Assoc* 1987; 257: 2591.
14. Kumana CR, Chau PY, Chan TK: Chloramphenicol use and childhood leukaemia. *Lancet* 1988; 1: 466.
15. Kumana CR, Ma J, Kung A, Kou M, Lauder: An assessment of drug information sheets for diabetic patients; only active involvement by patients is helpful. *Diabetes Research and Clinical Practice* 1988; 5: 225–231.
16. Kumana CR, Li KY, Chau PY: Worldwide variation in chloramphenicol utilisation: should it cause concern? *J Clin Pharmacol* 1988; 28(12).
17. Kumana CR, So SY, Li KY, Kou M and Chan SC: Pattern of anti-asthmatic drug utilization in Hong Kong compared to other parts of the world. *Resp Med* 1989 (in press).
18. Kumana CR, Li KY, Kou M and Chan SC: Cephalosporin and aminoglycoside utilisation in different parts of the world. *J Antimicrob Chemother* 1989 (in press).
19. Kumana CR: Antibiotic utilisation (Editorial). *J Am Med Assoc (SE Asia)* 1988; 4: 4–5.
20. Leung WHL, Lau JYN, Chan TK, Kumana CR: Fulminant hyperpyrexia induced by bleomycin. *Postgrad Med J* 1989; 417–419.
21. Kumana CR, Tse BSS, Chan YM, Kou M: Comparison of phenytoin bioavailability from dilantin (Parke-Davis) and a generic formulation from the PRC (used in HK government hospitals and clinics). *J HK Med Assoc* 1989 (in press).

Educational Articles on Clinical Pharmacology and Therapeutics (1983–1989)

1. Kumana CR: Drug treatment of epilepsy. *Hong Kong Practitioner* 1983; 5: 422–425.
2. Kumana CR, Tso SC, Yuen PM: Treatment of iron deficiency anaemia. *Hong Kong Practitioner* 1983; 5: 455–457.
3. Kumana CR, Wang R, Chen W: Beta blocking drugs and the prophylaxis of cardiovascular disease. *Hong Kong Practitooner* 1983; 5: 516–518.
4. Kumana CR, Lam Karen SL: Prescribing steroids. *Hong Kong Practitioner* 1983; 5: 702–706.
5. Kumana CR, So SY: The use of beta-adrenergic stimulation to produce bronchodilatation in asthma. *Hong Kong Practitioner* 1983; 5: 752–754.
6. Kumana CR, Chau PY: Cephalosporins. *Hong Kong Practitioner* 1984; 6: 941–947.
7. Kumana CR, Lam SK: Role of H$_2$ antagonists in the treatment and prevention of duodenal and gastric ulceration. *Hong Kong Practitioner* 1985; 7: 1291–1294.
8. Kumana CR, Stroebel AB, Mok CK: Antimicrobial chemoprophylaxis against infective endocarditis. *Hong Kong Practitioner* 1985; 7: 1342–1344.
9. Kumana CR, Yu YL, Richens A: Antiepileptic treatment during pregnancy. *J HK Med Assoc* 1985; 37: 98–99.
10. Kumana CR: Genuine advances in antimicrobial therapy. *J HK Med Assoc* 1985; 37: 148–151.
11. Kumana CR, Preston PJ & Arnold K: Drug prophylaxis of malaria. *J HK Med Assoc* 1985; 37: 195–198.
12. Kumana CR: An introduction to clinical pharmacology. *Hong Kong Practitioner* 1986; 8: 1881–1882.
13. Kumana CR, King NM, Li KY: Expoure of Hong Kong children to tetracyclines: a probable cause of widespread dental discolouration. *Hong Kong Practitioner* 1986; 8: 1938–1940.
14. Kumana CR, Chau PY, Todd D: How should we use cephalosporins. *Hong Kong Practitioner* 1986; 8: 2183–2186.
15. Kumana CR, Humphries M, Gabriel M: Clinical problems related to Anti-tuberculous drug therapy. *J HK Med Assoc* 1986; 38: 49–51.
16. Kumana CR: Hypertension and diabetes: the choice of antihypertensive therapy. *Hong Kong Practitioner* 1988; 10: 3551–3558.
19. Kumana CR and Chau PY: Choosing cephalosporins; which drug and when? *Med Progress* 1989; 16: 41–52.
20. Kumana CR, Chan MK: Drugs and renal disease, Part 1. *J HK Med Assoc* 1989 (in press).
21. Kumana CR, Chan MK: Drugs and renal disease, Part 2. *J HK Med Assoc* 1989 (in press).

C.R. KUMANA

ACHIEVEMENTS IN ENDOCRINOLOGY

In 1974, endocrinology was already an established discipline in the Department of Medicine. A metabolic ward and a hormone laboratory established in the early 1960s provided facilities for patient management, opportunities for training and stimulus for research. However, research efforts were mainly focused on carbohydrate metabolism and thyroid disorders. From 1974 to 1989, endocrinology in the Department of Medicine underwent considerable expansion and diversification. Research directions now include: carbohydrate metabolism, thyroid disorders, neuroendocrinology, metabolic bone diseases and reproductive endocrinology and infertility. Our role in patient care expanded from the original two clinics (diabetes and thyroid) in 1974 to the present of eight clinics including diabetes: general, home monitoring and gestational; thyroid; endocrine; osteoporosis; male infertility; and growth and puberty clinics. The latter two clinics are organized in conjunction with the Department of Obstetrics and Gynaecology and the Department of Paediatrics respectively. The team currently comprises 5 full time and 2 part time teachers, 2 registrars in training, 3 technical staff and 6 research assistants. The following is a brief description of the contributions of the endocrine division from 1974 to 1989.

Carbohydrate Metabolism

The department continued its efforts on the characterization of diabetes mellitus and its complications in the Chinese in Hong Kong (1–8). More recent studies showed a strong association of HLA DR3/DRw9 with insulin dependent diabetes mellitus (9). The department played a leading role in organizing education programmes for diabetic educators resulting in the establishment of diabetic nurses in major government hospitals.

The earlier description of hypoglycaemia associated with hepatocellular carcinoma was followed by studies on the mechanism causing the hypoglycaemia (10–12) as well as abnormalities in carbohydrate metabolism in post-necrotic cirrhosis of the liver (11, 13, 14). We also reported the occurrence of hypoglycaemia in patients with insulin autoimmunity (15). Studies of hypoglycaemia occurring in uraemic patients examined the changes in insulin, C-peptide and cyclic adenosine monophosphate levels as well as other metabolic substrates in these patients. These studies led to the finding of the important role of β adrenergic blockers in the generation of hypoglycaemia in haemodialysis patients (16–20).

Thyroid Diseases

The department was well known for its earlier study on the clinical features of thyrotoxic periodic paralysis and these were described in reviews and books (21, 22). The protective role of β adrenergic blocking agents in thyrotoxic periodic paralysis was further examined. Changes in the muscle calcium pump and erythrocyte sodium pump activities were observed (23, 24) and these shed some light on the pathogenesis and genetic basis of this common complication of thyrotoxicosis in the Orientals. Following the interest of the department in hypokalaemic periodic paralysis, the occurrence of this condition in association with primary hyperaldosteronism (25), renal tubular acidosis (26) and chronic ingestion of gossypol for contraception (27) were reported.

Studies on the changes in thyroid stimulating antibody activities in patients with thyrotoxicosis treated with antithyroid drugs, radioactive iodine, and subtotal thyroidectomy and in neonatal Graves' disease were fundamental in defining the role of immunoglobulins in the pathogenesis of thyrotoxicosis (28–31). Other studies described the incidence of hypothyroidism after radioactive iodine treatment of thyrotoxicosis (32) and acute myopathy in hypothyroidism (33). We also documented the association of HLA Bw46 in thyrotoxicosis (34, 35) and HLA DRw9 in Hashimoto's thyroiditis in Hong Kong (36).

In addition, we reported the effect of stress (37) and heroin addiction (38) on pituitary thyroid function; the determination of response of thyroid stimulating hormone and its α and β subunits to thyrotrophin releasing hormone in patients with various thyroid disorders (39); studies of thyroid hormone levels in patients with familial goitre due to organification defect (40); the regulation of carbohydrate and lipid metabolism in thyrotoxicosis (41, 42); and thyroid hyperfunction in trophoblastic diseases (43). The department was honoured when R Young was awarded the Daiichi-Mallinckrodt prize at the 4th Asia and Oceania Thyroid Association Meeting in 1989 in Seoul for her contribution to the field of thyroid diseases in this region.

Neuroendocrinology

Our clinical studies reported the usefulness of the dopamine agonist for the treatment of hyperprolactinaemia (44) and acromegaly (45). More recently we have reconfirmed the value of radiotherapy in acromegaly (46). We also studied and showed the effectiveness of a long acting somatostatin analogue in the treatment of acromegaly (47). In collaboration with the Department of Paediatrics we reported the long term use of pulsatile growth hormone releasing hormone therapy in children with growth hormone deficiency (48).

For the past 5 years, we have also focused our attention on the effects of cranial irradiation (for nasopharyngeal carcinoma) on the hypothalamic-pituitary axis. We reported the early occurrence of hypothalamic dysfunction after 2 years of cranial irradiation (49). These effects were progressive and hormone replacement was important in improving the quality of life of these patients with long-term survival after radiotherapy (50–52).

Basic research in neuroendocrinology started recently in the department on the regulation of vasoactive intestinal peptide and other related neuropeptides in the pituitary and hypothalamus. The level of the gene expression and post-translational processing of these peptides were regulated by thyroid hormones and oestrogens (53–55). This new area in basic neuroendocrinology is being actively pursued.

Calcium Homeostasis and Metabolic Bone Diseases

The department is currently involved in studies on osteoporosis in Chinese in Hong Kong with the goal of forming strategies and guidelines for the treatment of this condition. This ongoing clinical research showed that osteoporosis is common (56) and vitamin D deficiency is an important contributing factor in the pathogenesis of fracture neck of femur (57). The low intake of calcium in the Chinese diet in Hong Kong was documented (58, 59). The usefulness of intranasal calcitonin as an analgesic (60) and its bioavailability after intranasal administration were defined (61). With the recent availability of a dual energy X-ray bone absorptiometer, clinical studies with therapeutic intervention became possible in patients with high risks of developing osteoporosis such as post-menopausal women and hypogonadal patients.

The department embarked on basic science studies on the characterization of parathyroid hormone receptors in bone, kidney and skin fibroblasts in health and disease since 1987 (62–65). The occurrence and function of insulin receptors in osteoblasts were also examined (66). Recently clinical studies on parathyroid hormone like-protein occurring in hypercalcaemia of locally prevalent malignancies had begun (67).

Reproductive Endocrinology and Male Infertility

Clinical studies described the effects of various stresses, drugs and toxins on gonadal function including the effect of surgical stress (68), myocardial infarction (69), heroin addiction (70), cimetidine (71) and ranitidine (72). In addition, studies in collaboration with Professor David Todd reported the damaging effect of combination chemotherapy on gonadal function in patients with lymphoma and leukaemia (73, 74). More recently a longitudinal study demonstrated the presence of hypogonadotrophic hypogonadism in severe β thalassaemia and showed that chelation and pulsatile gonadotrophin-releasing hormone therapy were not useful in correcting gonadal dysfunction (75). The role of bioactive versus immunoreactive follicle stimulating hormone was also examined in patients with various gonadal dysfunction (76, 77).

In 1984, the male infertility clinic was established in collaboration with the Department of Obstetrics and Gynaecology. This clinic remained the only one of its kind in Hong Kong and served as a referral centre in the region. Together with the commitment to provide service, research on studies of various therapeutic regimens for male infertility was reported (78, 80). The results showed that in controlled studies many of the commonly used approaches (clomiphene and androgens) for infertile men with idiopathic oligospermia were of limited or no value. We also reported the low incidence of sino-pulmonary infections (81) and immunological dysfunction in patients with idiopathic oligospermia (82).

Recent studies focused on defining sperm function in normal and infertile men (83–94). The goal of these studies was to define parameters that might be of prognostic and predictive value in discriminating fertile from infertile men. Because of the active research in this area, the World Health Organization asked the department, together with the Departments of Obstetrics and Gynaecology and Physiology, to cohost an advanced workshop on sperm function in 1988, attended by participants from eleven countries.

The regulation of steroidogenesis and plasminogen activator production by granulosa cells of the ovary remained a long-term research focus. Studies demonstrated the role of trophic hormones on plasminogen activator production in the granulosa cells and its role in ovulation (95–99). More recently research expanded to examine the importance of tissue and urokinase-like plasminogen activators and their inhibitors in the same in vitro model (100).

Other Endocrine Disorders

As a referral centre for endocrine disorders in Hong Kong, we were fortunate to have the opportunity to observe, study and treat a large variety of patients with endocrine disorders. We studied, reported and contributed to the characterization of endocrine disease in this region. These include adrenal disorders: congenital adrenal hyperplasia due to 17α hydroxylase deficiency (101), Liddle's syndrome (102), primary hyperaldosteronism (25), Addison's disease in malignancy (103) and imaging of adrenal disorders (104); parathyroid tumours (105); precocious puberty (106); β sitosterolemia (107, 108), septo-optic dysplasia (109); insulinomas (12, 110); diabetes insipidus (111) among others.

Role in the Community and the Region

The department initiated and founded the Society for the Study of Endocrinology, Metabolism and Reproduction together with other members of the University. Through this local endocrine society the staff participated actively in open clinical meetings held both for the general practitioners and specialists on diverse subjects such as diabetes mellitus, thyroid disorders, growth problems and reproductive dysfunction.

Trainees from Australia, China, Philippines and the United States spent time in the laboratory and in the clinics sponsored by the China Medical Board, World Health Organization and Henry Luce Foundation. These fellows contributed to the research of the department. In 1986 members of the department organized and actively participated in a Postgraduate Course in Clinical Endocrinology held under the auspices of the Society for the Study of Endocrinology, Metabolism and Reproduction. This course was participated by clinicians from Australia, China, Malaysia, Philippines, Taiwan, Singapore, United Kingdom and United States in addition to Hong Kong. Members of the staff had been regularly invited to teach at post-graduate courses in endocrinology and reproductive medicine both in China and South East Asia.

The achievements in endocrinology in the Department of Medicine from 1974 to 1989 are possible through the continuous efforts of the endocrinologists including Drs. C.S. Teng and J. Ma who left but remained as honorary clinical lecturers; the early contributions of Dr. V. Chan; the capable and dedicated technicians, in particular P. Ho and A. Leung; the patience of our secretary, S. Yim; the dedication of the nurses of the metabolic ward E. Chan and G. Chan; the fellows and registrars who came and left; and the encouragement of our colleagues in the Department of Medicine led by Professor D. Todd.

References

1. Yeung RTT, Chan LKF: A study of diabetes mellitus among the Chinese in Hong Kong. In. *Proceedings of the Fifth Asia and Oceania Congress of Endocrinology. Chandigarh* (ed. Rastogi GK), Harmonic Printers, 1974; 2: 368–376.

2. Yeung RTT, Wang CCL, Chan LKF: The clinical and biochemical patterns of diabe-

tes mellitus in Hong Kong. In: *Diabetes Mellitus in Asia* (eds. Baba S, Goto Y, Fukui I), Excerpta Medica, Amsterdam, 1976; 131–136.

3. Yeung RTT: Treatment of diabetes mellitus in Southeast Asia. *Medical Progress* 1977; 4: 15–16.

4. Yeung RTT: Epidemiology of diabetes in Asia and Oceania. In: *Proceedings of 6th Asia and Oceania Congress of Endocrinology* (eds. Cheah JS, Lim P, Tambyah JA, Shanmugaratnam S, Yeo PPB, Ng CSA, Ng KKF), Stamford College Press, Singapore, 1978; 1: 217–226.

5. Yeung RTT, Wang C, Teng CS, Kwan S: The prevalence of cardiovascular complications in Chinese diabetic subjects. In: *Genetic Environmental Interaction in Diabetes Mellitus* (eds. Mellish JS, Hanna J, Baba S eds), Excerpta Medica, Amsterdam, 1981; ICS 549: 277–281.

6. Yeung RTT: Diabetes in S.E. Asia, viewpoint from Hong Kong. *Medical Progress* 1982; 9: 15–16.

7. Lam KSL, Ma JTC, Chan EYM, Yeung RTT: Sustained improvement in diabetic control in long-term self-monitoring of blood glucose. *Diabetes Res and Clin Practice* 1986; 2: 165–171.

8. Yeung RTT, Lam KSL, Ma JTC: Problems in the treatment of diabetes in in Hong Kong. In: *World Book of Diabetes in Practice* (ed. Krall L), Elsevier, Amsterdam, 1986; 2: 236–238.

9. Hawkins BR, Lam KSL, Ma JTC, Low LCK, Cheung PT, Sergeanbon SW, Yeung RTT: Strong association of HLA DR3/DRW9 heterozygosity with insulin dependent diabetes mellitus of early onset in Chinese. *Diabetes* 1987; 36: 1297–1300.

10. Pun KK, Ho PWM, Yeung RTT: Anomalous adenosine cyclic 3': 5'-monophosphate response to glucagon in patients with hepatocellular carinoma. *Cancer Res* 1986; 46: 2152–2154.

11. Pun KK, Ho PWM, Yeung RTT: C-peptide in non-alcoholic cirrhosis and hepatocellular carcinoma. *J Endocrinol Invest* 1988; 11: 337–343.

12. Pun KK, Young RTT, Wang C, Tam CF, Ho PWM: The use of glucagon challenge tests in the diagnostic evaluation of hypoglycae-

mia due to hepatoma, insulinoma and uraemia. *J Clin Endocrinol Metab* 1988; 67: 546–550.

13. Yeung RTT, Wang CCL: A study of carbohydrate metabolism in postnecrotic cirrhosis of liver. *Gut* 1974; 15: 907–912.

14. Teng CS, Ho P, Yeung RTT: Down-regulation of insulin receptors in post-necrotic cirrhosis of the liver. *J Clin Endocrinol Metab* 1982; 55: 524–533.

15. Benson EA, Ho P, Wang C, Wu PC, Fredland PN, Yeung RTT: Insulin autoimmunity as a cause of hypoglycaemia. *Arch Int Med* 1984; 144: 2351–2354.

16. Pun KK, Yeung CK, Ho PWM, Lin HJ, Chan MK, Yeung RTT: Effects of Propranolol and haemodialysis on the response of glucose, insulin, C-peptide and cyclic AMP to glucagon challenge. *Clin Nephrol* 1984; 21: 235–240.

17. Pun KK, Yeung CK, Yeung RTT: Effects of Propranolol and Metoprolol on glucose, cyclic AMP and insulin response during pharmacological hyperglucagonemia in hemodialysis patients. *Nephron* 1985; 39: 175–178.

18. Pun KK, Yeung CK, Yeung RTT: Propranolol-induced hypoglycaemia in a haemodialysis patient. *Dialysis and Transplantation* 1986; 15: 195–196.

19. Pun KK: Hypoglycaemia and insulin resistance in uraemia associated with insulin fragments. *Med Hypotheses* 1985; 17: 243–246.

20. Pun KK, Yeung CK, Chak W, Ho PWM, Chan MK, Lin HJ, Yeung RTT: Effects of selective and non-selective beta-blockers on alanine and free fatty acid responses to glucagon challenge in haemodialysis patients. *Clin Nephrol* 1986; 26(5): 222–226.

21. Yeung RTT: Thyroid disease in Southeast Asia. *Medical Progress* 1976; 3: 16–17.

22. Yeung RTT, Lam Karen SL: Thyroid disorders in the Far East. In: *Oxford Textbook of Medicine*, 2nd edition (eds. Weatherall DJ, Ledingham JGG, Warrell DA), Oxford Medical Publications, Oxford, 1987; 10.48–10.50.

23. Yeung RTT, Tse TF: Thyrotoxic periodic paralysis: Effect of propranolol. *Am J Med* 1974; 57: 584–590.

24. Lam KSL, Yeung RTT, Benson E, Wang C: Erythrocyte Na pump in thyrotoxic peri-

odic paralysis. *Aust NZ J Med* 1989; 19: 6–10.

25. Ma JTC, Wang C, Lam KSL, Yeung RTT, Chan FL, Boey J, Cheung PSY, Coghlan JP, Scoggins BA, Stockigt JR: A study of 50 consecutive patients with hyperaldosteronism in Hong Kong Chinese. *Q J Med* 1986; 61: 1021–1037.

26. Pun KK, Wong CK, Tsui E, Tam CF, Kung AWC, Wang C: Hypokalemic periodic paralysis due to Sjogren syndrome in Chinese patients. *Ann Intern Med* 1989; 110: 405–406.

27. Wang C, Yeung RTT: Gossypol and hypokalaemia. *Contraception* 1985; 32: 237–253.

28. Teng CS, Yeung RTT: Changes in thyroid-stimulating antibody activity in Graves' disease treated with antithyroid drug and its relationship to relapse: a prospective study. *J Clin Endocrinol Metab* 1980; 50: 144–147.

29. Teng CS, Yeung RTT, Khoo RKK, Alagaratnam TT: A prospective study of the changes in thyrotrophin-binding inhibitory immunoglobulins in Graves' disease treated by subtotal thyroidectomy or radioactive iodine. *J Clin Endocrinol Metab* 1980; 50: 1005–1010.

30. Teng CS, Tong TC, Hustchison JH, Yeung RTT: Thyroid-stimulating immunoglobulins in neonatal Graves' disease. *Arch Dis Child* 1980; 55: 894–895.

31. Teng CS, Yeung RTT, Kawa A, Nakamura S, Nomoto K, Arima N, Koreeda N, Tsuji K, Ho PWM: Thyrotrophin-binding inhibitory immunoglobulins and HLA-DRW3 — Two prognostic factors in Graves' disease. *Aust NZ J Med* 1981; 11: 383–385.

32. Best JD, Chan V, Khoo R, Teng CS, Wang C, Yeung RTT: Incidence of hypothyroidism after radioactive iodine therapy for thyrotoxicosis in Hong Kong Chinese. *Clin Radiol* 1981; 32: 57–61.

33. Kung AWC, Ma JTC, Yu YL, Wang C, Woo EKW, Lam KSL, Yeung RTT: Myopathy in acute hypothyroidism. *Postgrad Med J* 1987; 63: 661–663.

34. Hawkins BR, Ma JTC, Lam KSL, Wang CCL, Yeung RTT: Analysis of linkage between HLA haplotype and susceptibility to Graves' disease in multiple-case Chinese families in Hong Kong. *Acta Endocrinol* 1985; 110: 66–69.

35. Hawkins BR, Ma JTC, Lam KSL, Wang CCL,

Yeung RTT: Association of HLA antigens with thyrotoxic Graves' disease and periodic paralysis in Hong Kong Chinese. *Clin Endocrinol* 1985; 23: 245–252.

36. Hawkins BR, Lam KSL, Ma JTC, Wang C, Yeung RTT: Strong association between HLA-DRW9 and Hashimoto's thyroditis in Southern Chinese. *Acta Endocrinol* 1987; 114: 543–546.

37. Chan V, Wang C, Yeung RTT: Pituitary thyroid response to surgical stress. *Acta Endocrinol* 1978; 88: 490–498.

38. Chan V, Wang C, Yeung RTT: Effect of heroin addiction on thyrotropin, thyroid hormones and prolactin secretions in man. *Clin Endocrinol* 1979; 10: 557–565.

39. Chan V, Wang C, Yeung RTT: Thyrotropin, α, β subunits of thyrotropin and prolactin responses to 4-hour constant infusions of thyrotropin releasing hormone in normal subjects and patients with pituitary thyroid disorders. *J Clin Endocrinol Metab* 1979; 49: 127–131.

40. Chan V, Wang C, Yeung RTT: Dissociated thyroxine, triiodothyronine and reverse triiodothyronine levels in patients with familial goitre due to iodine organification defects. *Clin Endocrinol* 1979; 11: 257–265.

41. Lam KSL, Yeung RTT, Ho PWM, Lam SK: Glucose intolerance in thyrotoxicosis — role of insulin, glucagon and somatostain. *Acta Endocrinol* 1987; 114: 228–234.

42. Lam KSL, Yeung RTT, Chan MK: High–density lipoprotein cholesterol, hepatic lipase and lipoprotein lipase activities in thyroid dysfunction — effects of treatment. *Q J Med* 1986; 59: 513–521.

43. Chan V, Wang C, Ho PC, Yeung RTT, Ma HK: Biochemical thyroid hyperfunction in trophoblastic diseases. In: *Thyroid Research VIII* (eds. Stockigt JR, Nagataki S), Australian Academy of Science, Canberra, 1980; 598–601.

44. Wang C, Lam KSL, Ma JTC, Chan T, Liu MY, Yeung RTT: Long term treatment of hyperprolactinaemia with bromocriptine: effect of drug withdrawal. *Clin Endocrinol* 1987; 27: 363–372.

45. Wang C, Chan V, Yeung RTT: Treatment of acromegaly with Bromocriptine. *Aust NZ J Med* 1979; 9: 225–232.

46. Lam KSL, Wang C, Choi P, Ma JTC, Yeung

RTT: Long-term effects of megavoltage radiotherapy in acromegaly. *Aust NZ J Med* 1989; 19: 202–206.

47. Wang C, Lam KSL, Arceo E, Chan FL: Comparison of the effectiveness of subcutaneous injections every 8 hours versus every 2 hours of Somatostatin Analog (SMS 201–995) in the treatment of acromegaly. *J Clin Endocrinol Metab* 1989; 69: 670–677.

48. Low LCK, Wang C, Cheung PT, Ho P, Lam KSL, Yeung RTT, Yeung CY, Ling N: Long term pulsatile growth hormone releasing hormone therapy in children with growth hormone deficiency. *J Clin Endocrinol Metab* 1988; 66: 611–617.

49. Lam KSL, Wang C, Yeung RTT, Ma JTC, Tse VKC, Ho JHC: Early effects of cranial irradiation on hypothalamic pituitary function. *J Clin Endocrinol Metab* 1987; 64: 418–425.

50. Lam KSL, Wang C, Yeung RTT, Ma JTC, Ho JHC, Tse VKC, Ling N: Hypopituitarism following cranial irradiation for nasopharyngeal carcinoma. *Clin Endocrinol* 1986; 24: 643–651.

51. Lam KSL, Ho JHC, Lee AWM, Tse VKC, Chan PK, Wang C, Ma JTC, Yeung RTT: Symptomatic hypothalamic-pituitary dysfunction in nasopharyngeal carcinoma — Retrospective study. *Int J Radiat Oncol Biol Phys* 1987; 13: 1343–1350.

52. Woo E, Lam K, Yu YL, Ma J, Wang C, Yeung RTT: Temporal lobe and hypothalamic-pituitary dysfunction after radiotherapy for nasopharyngeal carcinoma — A distinct clinical syndrome. *J Neurol Neurosurg Psychiatry* 1988; 51: 1302–1307.

53. Lam KSL, Lechan RM, Segerson TP, Cacicedo L, Minamitani N, Reichlin S: Vasoactive intestinal peptide in the anterior pituitary is increased in hypothyroidism. *Endocrinology* 1989; 124: 1077–1084.

54. Lam KSL, Reichlin S: Pituitary vasoactive intestinal peptide is a paracrine regulator of prolactin release in the hypothyroid rat. *Neuroendocrinology* 1989 (in press).

55. Segerson TP, Lam KSL, Cacicedo L, Minamitani N, Fink S, Lechan RM, Reichlin S: Thyroid hormone regulates vasoactive intestinal peptide (VIP) mRNA levels in the rat anterior pituitary gland. *Endocrinology* 1989 (in press).

56. Pun KK, Yeung RTT: Osteoporosis — The silent epidemic. Editorial. SEA edition. *JAMA* 1988; 10: 506.

57. Pun KK: Importance of vitamin D deficiency among patients with fracture neck of femur in Hong Kong. *World Health Forum* (in press).

58. Pun KK, Chan LWL, Chung V, Wong FHW: Calcium and other dietary constituents in Hong Kong Chinese in relation to age and osteoporosis. *J Appl Nutrition* (in press).

59. Pun KK, Chan LWL, Chung V, Wong FHW: Calcium content of common food items in Chinese diet. *Calcif Tissue Int* (in press).

60. Pun KK, Chan LWL: The analgesic effect of intranasal salmon calcitonin in the treatment of osteoporotic vertebral fractures. *Clin Therapeutics* 1989; 11: 87–89.

61. Pun KK, Chan LWL, Lau P, Ho PWM and Wang C: Absorption of intranasal salmon calcitonin in normal subjects and hypogonadal men. *Calcif Tissue Int* 1989 (in press).

62. Pun KK, Ho PWM: Functional and structural characterization of the parathyroid hormone receptors on dog kidney, human kidney, chick bone and human dermal fibroblast: a comparative study of the homologous functional and structural properties. *Biochem J* 1989; 259: 785–789.

63. Pun KK, Ho PWM: Parathyroid hormone inhibits collagen synthesis and mitogenesis of clonal rat osteoblastic cell line UMR-106. *J Biochem* (in press).

64. Pun KK, Ho PWM, Nissenson RA: Desensitization of parathyroid hormone receptors on cultured bone cells. *J Bone Mineral Research* (in press).

65. Pun KK, Ho PWM, Lau P: Effects of aluminium on the parathyroid hormone receptors of bone and kidney. *Kidney Int* (in press).

66. Pun KK, Ho PWM, Lau P: The regulation and function of insulin receptors on an osteosarcoma cell line. *J Bone Mineral Research* 1989 (in press).

67. Buday AA, Nissenson RA, Klein RF, Pun KK, Clark OH, Diep D, Aranud CD, Strewler GJ: Increased serum levels of a parathyroid hormone-like protein in malignancy-associated hypercalcaemia. *Ann Intern Med* (in press).

68. Wang C, Chan V, Yeung RTT: Effect of sur-

gical stress of pituitary-testicular function. *Clin Endocrinol* 1978; 9: 255–266.

69. Wang C, Chan V, Yeung RTT: Effect of acute myocardial infarction on pituitary-testicular function. *Clin Endocrinol* 1978; 9: 249–254.

70. Wang C, Chan V, Yeung RTT: The effect of heroin addiction on pituitary-testicular function. *Clin Endocrinol* 1978; 9: 455–462.

71. Wang C, Lai CL, Lam KC, Yeung KK: Effect of cimetidine on gonadal function in man. *Br J Clin Pharmacol* 1982; 13: 791–794.

72. Wang C, Wong KL, Lam KC, Lai CL: Ranitidine does not affect gonadal function in men. *Br J Clin Pharmacol* 1983; 16: 430–432.

73. Wang C, Ng RP, Chan TK, Todd D: Effect of combination chemotherapy in pituitary-gonadal function in patients with lymphoma and leukemia. *Cancer* 1980; 45: 2030–2037.

74. Wang C, Ng RP, Chan TK, Todd D: Leydig cell dysfunction after combination chemotherapy. *Lancet* 1981; ii: 529.

75. Wang C, Tso SC, Todd D: Hypogonadotropic hypogonadism in severe β-thalassemia: effect of chelation and pulsatile gonadotropin-releasing hormone therapy. *J Clin Endocrinol Metab* 1989; 68: 511–516.

76. Wang C, Dahl KD, Leung A, Chan SYW, Hsueh AJW: Serum bioactive follicle stimulating hormone in men with idiopathic oligospermia. *J Clin Endocrinol Metab* 1987; 65: 629–633.

77. Wang C: Bioassays of follicle-stimulating hormone. *Endocrine Reviews* 1988; 9: 374–377.

78. Wang C, Chan CW, Wong KK, Yeung KK: Comparison of the effectiveness of placebo, clomiphene citrate, mesterolone, pentoxifylline and testosterone rebound therapy for the treatment of idiopathic oligospermia. *Fertil Steril* 1983; 40: 358–365.

79. Wang C, Chan SYW, Tang LCH, Yeung KK: Clomiphene citrate does not improve spermatozoal fertilizing capacity in idiopathic oligospermia. *Fertil Steril* 1985; 44: 102–105.

80. Chan SYW, Wang CCL, Tang LCH: Effect of clomiphene citrate (CC) on human spermatozoal motility and fertility capacity in vitro. *Fertil Steril* 1985; 43: 773–776.

81. Wang C, So SY, Wong KK, So WWK, Chan SYW: Chronic sinopulmonary disease in Chinese patients with obstructive azoospermia. *J Andrology* 1987; 8: 225–229.

82. Zhong CQ, Ho PC, Fan MC, Chan SYW, So WWK, Wang C: Immunological studies in patients with oligospermia. *Fertil Steril* (in press).

83. Wang C, Chan SYW, Leung A, Ng RP, Ng M, Tang LCH, Ma HK, Tsoi WL, Kwan M: Cross-sectional study of semen parameters in a large group of normal Chinese men. *Int J Andrology* 1985; 8: 257–274.

84. Chan SYW, Fox EJ, Tang LCH, Chan MC, Tsoi WL, Wang C, Tang GWK, Ho PC: The relationship between the human spermatozoa hypo-osmotic swelling test and the human spermatozoa zona-free hamster ova penetration assay. *Fertil Steril* 1985; 44: 668–672.

85. Chan SYW, Loh TT, Wang C, Tang LCH: Seminal plasma transferrin and seminiferous tubular dysfunction. *Fertil Steril* 1986; 46: 687–691.

86. Chan SYW, Wang C: Correlation between semen adenosine triphosphate (ATP) and sperm fertilizing capacity. *Fertil Steril* 1987; 47: 717–719.

87. Chan SYW, Li SQ, Wang C: Test egg yolk buffer storage increases the human sperm fertlizing capacity. *Int J Andrology* 1987; 10: 517–524.

88. Chan SYW, Wang C, Ng M, So WWK, Ho PC: Multivariate discriminant analysis on the relationship between the human sperm hypoosmotic swelling test and the human sperm in vitro fertilizing capacity. *Int J Andrology* 1988; 11: 369–378.

89. Wang C, Chan SYW, Ng M, So WWK, Tsoi WL, Lo T, Leung A: Diagnostic value of sperm function tests and routine semen analyses in fertile and infertile men. *J Andrology* 1988; 9: 384–389.

90. Chan SYW, Wang C, Ng M, Tam G, Lo T, Tsoi WL, Nie G, Leung J: Evaluation of computerized analysis of sperm movement characteristics and differential sperm tail swelling patterns in predicting human sperm in vitro fertilizing capacity. *J Andrology* 1989; 10: 133–138.

91. Chan SYW, Wang C, Chan STH, Ho PC, So WWK, Chan YF, Ma HK: Predictive value of sperm morphology and movement characteristics in the outcome of in vitro fertili-

zation of human oocytes. *J In Vitro Fertilization and Embryo Transfer* 1989 (in press).

92. Chan SYW, Wang C, Song BL, Lo T, Leung A, Tsoi WL, Leung J: Computer assisted image analysis of sperm concentration in human semen before and after swim-up separation — Comparison with haemocytometer assessment. *Int J Andrology* 1989; (in press).

93. Chan SYW, Zhang GH, Leung A, Ng M, Wang C: Evaluation of the semi-automated autosperm semen analysis system II Comparison with conventional method, time exposure photomicrography and automated Cellsoft system. *Fertil Steril* 1989 (in press).

94. Chan SYW, Wang C, Chan STH, Ho PC, So WWK, Chan YF: Differential evaluation of human sperm hypoosmotic swelling test and its effect on the outcome of in vitro fertilization of human oocytes. *Human Reproduction* 1989 (in press).

95. Wang C, Chan V: Divergent effects of prolactin on estrogen and progesterone production by granulosa cells of rat ovarian follicles. *Endocrinology* 1982; 110: 1085–1093.

96. Wang C: Luteinizing hormone releasing hormone stimulates plasminogen activator production by rat granulosa cells. *Endocrinology* 1983; 112: 1130–1132.

97. Wang C, Leung A: Gonadotropins regulate plasminogen activator production by rat granulosa cells. *Endocrinology* 1983; 112: 1201–1207.

98. Wang C, Leung A: LHRH stimulates plasminogen activator and inhibits steroid production by granulosa cells of adult rat Graafian follicles. *Mol Cell Endocrinol* 1986; 44: 61–68.

99. Wang C, Leung A: Estrogens, progestogens, and androgens enhance the follicle stimulating hormone stimulated plasminogen activator production by rat granulosa cells. *Endocrinology* 1987; 120: 2131–2136.

100. Wang C, Leung A: Glucocorticoids stimulate plasminogen activator production by rat granulosa cells. *Endocrinology* 1989; 124: 1595–1601.

101. Wang C, Yeung RTT, Coghlan JP, Oddie CJ, Scoggins BA, Stockigt JR: Hypertension due to 17α-hydroxylase deficiency. *Aust NZ J Med* 1978; 8: 296–299.

102. Wang C, Chan TK, Yeung RTT, Coghlan JP, Scoggins BA, Stockigt JR: The effect of triamterene and sodium intake on renin, aldosterone, and erythrocyte sodium transport in Liddle's Syndrome. *J Clin Endocrinol Metab* 1981; 52: 1027–1032.

103. Kung AWC, Pun KK, Lam Karen SL, Wang C, Leung CY: Addisonian crisis as presenting feature in malignancy. *Cancer* (in press).

104. Chan FL, Wang C: Imaging for adrenal tumours. In: *Imaging Endocrine Disorders. Baillier's Clinical Endocrinology and Metabolism* (eds. Chan FL, Wang C), Balliere Tindal, London, 1989; 3: 153–189.

105. Cheung PSY, Boey JH, Wang CCL, Ma JTC, Lam KSL, Yeung RTT: Primary hyperparathyroidism — Its clinical pattern and results of surgical treatment in Hong Kong Chinese. *Surgery* 1988; 103: 558–562.

106. Low LCK, Cheung PT, Wang C, Chan FL: Long term treatment of precocious puberty using an intranasal luteinizing hormone releasing hormone analog (Buserelin). *Aust J Paediatr* (in press).

107. Wang C, Lin HJ, Chan TK, Salen G, Chan WC, Tse TF: A unique patient with coexisting cerebrotendinous xanthomatosis and β-sitosterolemia. *Am J Med* 1981; 71: 313–319.

108. Lin HJ, Wang C, Salen G, Lam KC, Chan TK: Sitosterol and cholesterol metabolism in a patient with coexisting phytosterolemia and cholestanolemia. *Metabolism* 1983; 32: 126–133.

109. Lam KSL, Wang C, Ma JTC, Leung SP, Yeung RTT: Hypothalamic defects in two adult patients with septo-optic dysplasia. *Acta Endocrinol* 1986; 112: 305–309.

110. Kung AWC, Ma John TC, Wang C, Fu KH, Lam KSL, Yeung RTT: Prevention of hypoglycaemia in a patient with pancreatic microadenomatosis by a long-acting somatostatin analogue SMS 201-995. *Clin Endocrinol* 1987; 27: 469–473.

111. Pun KK, Chan G, Wang C, Yeung RTT: Cranial diabetes insipidus presenting as pyrexia of undetermined origin. *Am J Med* 1989; 86: 732–733.

R.T.T. YOUNG, Christina WANG,
K.S.L. LAM, K.K. PUN and A.W.C. KUNG

Research in Gastroenterology

A combined gastrointestinal unit has been set up between the University Departments of Medicine and Surgery since the years of Prof. McFadzean, including a combined ward and a combined gastrointestinal clinic. The combined approach has provided a strong basis for intense basic and clinical research programmes, good-quality under- and post-graduate training, and consequently high-standard, peer-reviewed patient-care. The medical and surgical team has since each subspecialized into solid organ and the lumen, namely hepatology and gastroenterology, following international trends. The Department of Medicine has pioneered the development and training of gastrointestinal endoscopy in Hong Kong. For example, diagnostic and therapeutic ERCP has been a routine since 1975 and endoscopic haemostasis and cancer vaporization by laser, bicap and heater-probe since 1985. The gastroenterological setup and endoscopy service has attracted many individually and institutionally based trainees, local and abroad, to join the tightly scheduled training programmes that have been running over the past 15 years.

PEPTIC ULCER

Concept of Heterogeneity

It is proposed that not only is duodenal ulcer a different disease from gastric ulcer as has been classically established, but that each in itself is heterogeneous in origin (1). This is supported by observations made clinically (2–6), genetically (3, 7–10), and pathophysiologically (11–25). This concept is now generally accepted and has been helpful for the understanding of the aetiology, prognostic factors, and responses to various forms of treatment of peptic ulcer.

Early- and Late-onset Duodenal Ulcer

Approximately 50% of duodenal ulcer patients whose symptoms begin before the age of 30 (early-onset) have a positive history of familial ulcer dyspepsia, whereas only 20% of those whose symptoms start after the age of 30 (late-onset) have such a history. Late-onset patients have blood group O prevalence, whereas the blood group distribution in early-onset patients is similar to the general population. This is true in Hong Kong (3), and has been shown in western countries such as Scotland and Czechoslovakia. Significantly more males, more acid hypersecretors and more gastrointestinal bleeding are found amongst early-onset patients than in late-onset patients (4). There is a significantly increased tendency for the late-onset ulcers to perforate, to become stenosed, to have severe exacerbation, and to be virulent — that is, to be multiple, post-bulbar or giant (3). Two subgroups of early-onset familial duodenal ulcer patients have been identified, one having possible G cell hyperfunction and the other parietal cell hyperfunction (7).

Parietal Cell Mass and Maximal Acid Output

There is a large ethnic difference in the size of the parietal cell mass between Caucasian and Chinese patients with duodenal ulcer, that of the Scots, for example, being almost double that of the Chinese, and this remains true after correction for differences in body weight (10, 25). This has important therapeutic implications when selecting the appropriate dosage of antisecretary agents for the Chinese patients. The dosage of antacids, cimetidine, and omeprazole has been found to be smaller than that used in Caucasian patients (26–28).

In all countries studied, a significant proportion of duodenal ulcer patients have abnormally large maximal acid output (following maximal stimulation with usually pentagastrin), and this proportion varies from 20% to 50% (22); about one-third of duodenal ulcer patients in Hong Kong belong to this group of hypersecretors (16).

Basal Acid Secretion

Basal acid output and acid response to cephalic stimulation (sight, smell and taste) is generally taken to reflect the vagal drive on the stomach. The proportion of duodenal ulcer patients with abnormally high basal output varies between 10–20% and about 10% of Chinese patients in Hong Kong have this abnormality (22). About one-third of patients with duodenal ulcer have increased cephalic acid output (11, 12).

Sensitivity of Parietal Cells to Gastrin

Interestingly, patients with duodenal ulcer may have increased sensitivity to the stimulation by endogenous gastrin secreted in response to meals, and consequently secretes a larger amount of acid after meals (15). About 25% of Hong Kong patients have increased sensitivity to gastrin (29).

Gastrin and Somatostatin

We developed one of the earliest radioimmunoassays on gastrin and somatostatin (13, 30–32). About one-third of patients with duodenal ulcer have abnormally high gastrin secretion following meals (8), and this abnormality occurs commonly in patients with normal acid secretion (13), a finding confirmed by a number of investigators as has been reviewed (33). Meal-stimulated gastrin secretion may also be inappropriately high relative to the sensitivity of their parietal cells to gastrin (18). Patients with duodenal ulcer have high post-prandial somatostatin, which is most likely a secondary phenomenon (32).

Of the three types of gastric ulcer, corpus ulcers are associated with low acid and high gastrin, whereas prepyloric ulcers are associated with high acid and low gastrin, reflecting the degree of body gastritis; gastric ulcers associated with duodenal ulcer are associated with high gastrin

and high acid, suggesting that high gastrin plays a dominant pathophysiological role (19).

Gastric Emptying

Abnormally increased gastric emptying may lead to increased duodenal acid load. A defect in slowing gastric emptying in the face of increasing duodenal acid load has been demonstrated in patients with duodenal ulcer (17).

Serum Pepsinogen I and II

Hyperpepsinogenaemia I occurs in duodenal ulcer patients as a group and is a known genetic marker of the condition. It occurs in 36% of Chinese patients, and there is no difference in pepsinogen I and II levels, and in the pepsinogen I: II ratio that reflects histological gastritis, between Chinese and American, both in normal controls and ulcer patients (34).

Histamine and Enterochromaffin-like (ECL) Cells

It is well known that histamine stimulates acid secretion through H2-receptors. The source of histamine in the human stomach, however, is not known. Using a specific histochemical method, the source of histamine has recently been located to the ECL cells, which are paracrine cells situated in the neighbourhood of the parietal cells and they receive cholinergic nerve supply (35, 36). This exciting finding raises many questions, the foremost of which is whether duodenal ulcer patients have an increased number of ECL cells.

Campylobacter Pylori

Many studies including our own (37, 38) have observed a close association of this organism, found mostly in the antrum of the stomach, with antral gastritis and peptic ulceration. Does it cause peptic ulcer? Despite healing of duodenal or gastric ulcer, whether this occurs naturally with the use of placebo (37) or therapeutically following active treatment (37–39), these organisms persist in the stomach. They persist and remain unchanged during the time of remission and at subsequent ulcer relapse (40). These studies speak against a pathophysiological role.

Meal-stimulated and Nocturnal Acid Secretion

As can be seen from the above, there are many physiological abnormalities in peptic ulcer disease. It is not known how these abnormalities are distributed in a given population of patients. However, the abnormalities described in duodenal ulcer, either alone or in combination, can theoretically lead to an increased meal-stimulated acid secretion, since this represents a common pathway for the various abnormal mechanisms of acid secretion. Another common pathway is possibly the nocturnal acid secretion. A review of the literature indeed shows that an increased meal-stimulated acid secretion or an increased nocturnal acid secretion can each be demonstrated in about 60% of patients (22).

Epidemiology

Hong Kong is the only place in the world where the incidence of peptic ulcer manifests an increasing trend (41). It has long been suspected that geographical variation in incidence of peptic ulcer occurs (42), but direct comparison between countries has not been performed. A collaborative study with Australia shows that perforated peptic ulcer is five times more common in Hong Kong than in Sydney, that perforated duodenal ulcer is 15 times more common in Hong Kong, a result possibly of society stress, and that perforated gastric ulcer is three times more common in Australia, a result possibly of habitual use of analgesics by the Australians (43). Examining the perforation rates in Hong Kong over the past 25 years shows a strong correlation with society stress (44). Seasonal variation in ulcer incidence is known to occur; in Hong Kong, the peak occurs in November and December (45).

Treatment of Peptic Ulcer

Can duodenal ulcer be effectively healed by controlling meal-stimulated acid secretion?

Taking two antacid tablets 1 and 3 h after meals and nocte (neutralizing capacity of 175 mmol HCl per day) heals 70% of duodenal ulcers in 4 wk compared with 33% when placebos are used (26). This study has since been confirmed by no less than 10 other reports as has recently been reviewed (46–49), leaving little doubt that controlling acid secretion in response to meals is effective for the healing of duodenal ulcer.

Can Duodenal Ulcer be Effectively Healed by Controlling Nocturnal Acid Secretion?

A pioneering placebo-controlled study in Hong Kong shows that a single dose of H_2-receptor antagonist (oxmetidine) taken at bedtime effectively heals about 70% of duodenal ulcer (50). This observation has since been supported by other studies including our own (51) that compare nocturnal dosing of H_2-receptor antagonists with other established dosage schemes for these agents, as has been reviewed (24, 52).

Which is More Important — Controlling Day time Meal-stimulated Acid Secretion or Nocturnal Acid Secretion?

Comparing three cimetidine regimens: (i) 400 mg tds with meals, (ii) 1200 mg at bedtime, and (iii) a reference regimen using the same total daily dose in the form of 200 mg tds and 600 mg bedtime, shows that the healing efficacy is significantly better with the meal-time regimen than the other two, and this is attributable to a faster healing at 2 wk (53). This study shows that in the planning of an acid-reducing regemen for duodenal ulcer, the meal-time acid secretion cannot be ignored. This conforms with the recent observations including our own that the use of omeprazole, a proton pump inhibitor that suppresses acid production significantly greater than H_2-receptor antagonists (54) and significantly controls both day-time and night-time acid secretion, heals duodenal ulcer significantly faster than H_2-receptor antagonists (55, 56).

Do Cytoprotective Mechanisms Heal Ulcer?

These mechanisms, which include mucus and

bicarbonate secretion, restitution and prolongation of epithelial cells, and improvement of microcirculation (57), protect gastric mucosa from injuries such as those due to ethanol and nonsteroidal anti-inflammatory agents. These are classical actions of the E-type prostaglandins. Can they be made use of to heal ulcers?

E-prostaglandins

Interestingly, prostaglandin is the first agent shown to improve antral gastritis (58). A number of studies including our own (59, 60) have shown that misoprostol and enprostil, the two available oral preparations of E-type prostaglandins, are able to heal duodenal and gastric ulcers, as has recently been reviewed (61–66). Diarrhoea appears to be a common side effect of prostaglandin among Chinese (59).

Site-protective agents

Tripotassium dicitrato bismuthate (TDB). This has been shown to adhere biochemically to the base of experimental ulcers for at least 6 h, thereby forming a mechanical layer that protects the ulcer base from the luminal acid and pepsin, and attracting large numbers of macrophages, which are presumably healing forces, to the ulcer site (67). There is preliminary evidence that TDB may be cytoprotective, good evidence that it is bacteriocidal to Campylobacter pylori, and strong evidence that it heals duodenal and gastric ulcers (61, 63, 64, 68–70).

Sucralfate. Sucralfate has similar site-protective properties and well defined cytoprotective mechanisms (71, 72). It has recently been shown to be a potent agent in improving the gastric microcirculation (73). It has led to the discovery that cytoprotective mechanisms can be prostaglandin dependent and prostaglandin independent (74). Like prostaglandin, sucralfate effectively improves histological antral gastritis (75). Like H_2-receptor antagonists, it heals about 70% of duodenal ulcers in 4 wk (76) and 70% of gastric ulcers in 8 wk (77). These observations strongly suggest that cytoprotective mechanisms *per se* are able to heal ulcers.

Does Ulcer Healing by Acid-reduction Differ from That by Cytoprotective Mechanisms?

Cigarette smoking. We have shown that cigarette smoking impairs healing of duodenal ulcer by placebo, antacids (26), H_2-receptor antagonists (78) and omeprazole (55), as has recently been reviewed (79). We have observed, interestingly, that healing by prostaglandin (59), colloidal bismuth (69), and sucralfate (76) is unaffected by cigarette smoking. Supportive evidence is available in the literature, as has been reviewed recently (80).

Refractory ulcer. Duodenal ulcer refractory to H_2-receptor antagonists can be effectively treated with colloidal bismuth (81)and possibly with sucralfate (76). These findings have been confirmed, as reviewed recently (82), and suggest different underlying pathophysiology for such ulcers.

Ulcer relapse. Duodenal ulcers treated initially with sucralfate relapse later than ulcers treated initially with H_2-receptor antagonists (76). Similar findings have been reported by other investigators and also with the use of cytoprotective agents such as colloidal bismuth, carbenoxolone sodium and anti-cholinergics, as has recently been reviewed (83). These observations can be explained if cytoprotective agents lead to 'better' healing or if acid-reducing agents lead to up-regulation or increase in sensitivity of the parietal cells. Evidence for both is available (84).

Which Form of Ulcer Surgery?

In a prospective study comparing proximal gastric vagotomy (PGV), truncal vagotomy and drainage, and truncal vagotomy and antrectomy, it has been observed that the severer form of surgery has lesser recurrence but higher morbidity and mortality, and the recurrent rate after PGV is 16% at 12 mo (85). Recurrence following surgery can be successfully treated with H_2-receptor antagonists (86) and colloidal bismuth (68). The best predictive factors of recurrence are based on both acid secretions and clinical history (87–89).

Which Therapeutic Endoscopy Method for Bleeding Ulcer?

A randomized comparative study on patients with actively bleeding peptic ulcer as demonstrated by endoscopy shows that LASER, bipolar electrical, and heater-probe coagulation are equally effective, achieving haeostasis in 89–96% of patients. Heater-probe costs HK$400 per patient, whereas LASER costs HK$1600 (90).

What are the Prognostic Factors for Ulcer Healing?

In our experience, the most consistently observed factors that predict failure to heal by acid-reducing agents include cigarette smoking, long-standing symptoms, hyperacidity, and duodenal bulb deformity, as has been reviewed (52, 79, 80, 82, 83). Genetic factors as evident by hyperpepsinogenaemia I appears also to play a part in the Chinese community (91).

Which is the Most Appropriate Form of Maintenance Therapy?

Of 8 regimens of maintenance treatment randomly given to about 800 patients with duodenal ulcer for one year, antacid tablets ii tds, cimetidine 400 mg nocte, ranitidine 150 mg nocte, and sucralfate 1 g bd were found to be equally effective; trimipramine and pirenzepine were ineffective. Antacid is associated with the highest frequency of side effects (92).

GASTRITIS

Acute Gastritis

A laser-doppler technique of measuring relative gastric mucosal blood flow, and a hydrogen clearance method of measuring the absolute flow have been developed (93) and verified (73) to study the relationship of the gastric microcirculation and experimental gastritis. Ethanol reduces blood flow and causes mucosal damage, and nicotine potentiates these effects; both are preventable by sucralfate (94) and zinc sulphate (95). Superficial gastritis due to acute stress in rats is related to reduction of mucosal blood flow (96). Misoprostol (prostaglandin E1) and sucralfate dose-dependently, and omeprazol at high dose, increase mucosal blood flow; interestingly, sucralfate achieves the highest flow (73, 97). The effect of sucralfate on blood flow cannot be obtained by individual components of sucralfate including aluminium, and requires the whole sucralfate molecule (98).

Chronic Gastritis

Antral gastritis, Campylobacter pylori and peptic ulcer are closely related (99). Antral gastritis associated with duodenal ulcer can be effectively improved by misoprostol (58), sucralfate (75), and omeprazole (100), and the effect is independent on ulcer healing. These agents have no antibacterial effect on Campylobacter pylori. The clinical significance of this improvement is not known, and appears unrelated to subsequent relapse.

About 50% of patients with non-ulcer dyspepsia have histological antral gastritis and 50% have abnormal gastroduodenal motility pattern, but the overlap is unknown (99). 80% of patients with non-ulcer dyspepsia respond symptomatically to sulpiride, a dopamine antagonist that improves gastric emptying (101).

RECURRENT PYOGENIC CHOLANGITIS

Endoscopic retrograde cholangiopancreatography (ERCP) offers accurate assessment of this condition and helps the planning of subsequent management (102). It reveals that gall stones occur in about one-third of these patients and that clonorchiasis occurs in about one-fifth. Clonorchis probably plays a secondary role in recurrent pyogenic cholangitis (103). Endoscopic sphincterotomy is safe even in the old and frail, and effective in over 90% of patients with stones confined to the common bile duct. Permanent internal drainage can be established and re-stenosis of the papillotomy site is rare (104). This has become standard treatment since 1976, and has clear advantages over surgery in patients with stones in the common bile duct (105).

References

1.   Lam SK: Clinical and pathophysiological studies on duodenal ulceration: evidence

for the existence of two populations. MD Thesis, University of Hong Kong, 1975.

2.   Lam SK, Sircus W: Studies on duodenal ulcer I. The clinical evidence for the existence of two populations. *Q J Med* 1975; 44: 369–387.

3.   Lam SK, Ong GB: Duodenal ulcers: early and late onset. *Gut* 1976; 17: 169–179.

4.   Lam SK, Koo J, Sircus W: Early and late onset duodenal ulcers in Chinese and Scots. *Scand J Gastroenterol* 1983; 18: 651–658.

5.   Hui WM, Lam SK: Multiple duodenal ulcer. *Gut* 1987; 28: 1134–1141.

6.   Lam SK, Chan PKW, Cheng FCY, Ong GB: The inter-relationship between bleeding, perforation and stenosis in duodenal ulceration. *Aust NZ J Surg* 1978; 4: 152–155.

7.   Lam SK, Ong GB: Identification of two subgroups of familial early onset duodenal ulcers. *Ann Int Med* 1980; 93: 540–544.

8.   Lam SK, Ong GB: Relationship of postprandial serum gastrin response to sex, body weight, blood group status, familial dys pepsia, duration and age of onset of ulcer symptoms in duodenal ulcer. *Gut* 1980; 21: 528–532.

9.   Lam SK, Hui KK, Ho J, Wong KP, Rotters JI, Samloff MI: Pachy-dermoperiostosis and peptic ulcer. *Gastroenterology* 1983; 84: 834–839.

10.   Prescott RJ, Lam SK, Hasan M, Sircus W, Wong J, Ong GB: The relationship between body parameters and gastric acid secretion in normal controls and duodenal ulcer subjects in two ethnic groups. *Italian J Gastroenterol* 1980; 12: 167–170.

11.   Lam SK, Sircus W: Vagal hyperactivity in duodenal ulcers: with and without acid hypersecretion. *Rendiconti Gastroenterol* 1975;7: 5–8.

12.   Lam SK, Sircus W: A comparison of the acid and gastrin secretory response to hypoglycaemia and meals in duodenal ulcer with and without acid hypersecretion to pentagastrin. *Digestion* 1976; 14: 1–11.

13.   Byrnes DJ, Lam SK, Sircus W: The relation between functioning parietal cell and gastrin cell masses in two groups of duodenal ulcer patients. *Clin Sci Mol Med* 1976; 50: 375–383.

14.   Lam SK, Sircus W: Cholinergic suppression of the acid response to pentagastrin in normosecreting and hypersecreting duodenal ulcer patients. *Rendiconte Gastroenterol* 1977; 9: 9–12.

15.   Lam SK, Isenberg JI, Grossman MI, Lane WH, Walsh JH: Gastric acid secretion is abnormally sensitive to meal-stimulated endogenous gastrin in duodenal ulcer patients. *J Clin Invest* 1980; 65: 555–562.

16.   Lam SK, Hasan M, Sircus W, Wong J, Ong GB, Prescott RJ: A comparison of the maximal acid output and gastrin response to meals in Chinese and Scots, normals and with duodenal ulcer. *Gut* 1980; 21: 324–328.

17.   Lam SK, Isenberg JI, Grossman MI, Hogan D, Lane WH: Rapid gastric emptying in duodenal ulcer. *Dig Dis Sci* 1982; 27: 598–604.

18.   Walsh JH, Lam SK, Isenberg JI: Autoregulation of gastrin release in duodenal ulcer disease. In: *Gut Peptides and Ulcer* (ed. Miyoshi A), Biomedical Research Foundation, Tokyo, 1983; pp. 280–283.

19.   Lam SK, Lai CL: Gastric ulcers with and without associated duodenal ulcer have different pathophysiology. *Clin Sci Mol Med* 1978; 55: 97–102.

20.   Lam SK: Physiologic abnormalities and heterogeneity of peptic ulcer. In: *International Workshop on Genetics and Heterogeneity of Common Gastrointestinal Disorders* (eds. Rotter JI, Samloff IM and Rimoin DL), Academic Press, New York, London, Toronto, Sydney, San Francisco, 1982; pp. 67–80.

21.   Lam SK: Heterogeneous origin of hyperacidity in duodenal ulcer. In: *Workshop on Genetic and Clinical Aspects of Pepsinogen* (eds. Kreuning J, Meuwissen SGM, Eriksson AW), 1985; pp. 255–271.

22.   Lam SK: Pathogenesis and pathophysiology of duodenal ulcer. In: *Peptic Ulcer Disease. Clinics in Gastroenterology* (eds. Isenberg JI, Johanssen C), WB Saunders, London, Philadelphia, Toronto, 1984; 13: 447–472.

23.   Lam SK: Aetiology of gastric and duodenal ulcer. In: *Annals of the Academy of Medicine, Singapore* (ed. LaBrooy S), 1983; 12: 498–506.

24.   Lam SK, Hui WM, Ng MTT: The stomach. In: *Current Gastroenterology* (ed. Gitnick GL), Year Book Medical Publishers, Chi-

cago, London, 1987; pp. 31–65.

25. Cheng FCY, Lam SK, Ong GB: Maximum acid output to graded doses of pentagastrin and its relation to parietal cell mass in Chinese patients with duodenal ulcer. *Gut* 1977; 18: 827–832.

26. Lam SK, Lam KC, Lai CL, Yeung CK, Yam LYC, Wong WS: Treatment of duodenal ulcer with antacid and sulpiride — A double blind con trolled study. *Gastroenterology* 1979; 76: 315–322.

27. Lam SK, Koo J: Accurate prediction of duodenal-ulcer healing rate by discriminant analysis. *Gastroenterology* 1983; 85: 403-13-12.

28. Hui WM, Lam SK, Lau WY, Branicki FJ, Lok ASF, Ng MMT, Lai CL, Poon GP: Omeprazole and ranitidine in duodenal ulcer healing and subsequent relapse — A randomized double-blind study with weekly endoscopic assessment. *J Gastroenterol Hepatol* 1989 (in press).

29. Lam SK, Koo J: Gastrin sensitivity in duodenal ulcer. *Gut* 1985; 26: 485–490.

30. Lam SK, Lai CL: Inhibition of sulpiride on the cephalic phase of gastric acid and gastrin secretion in duodenal ulcer patients. *Scand J Gastroenterol* 1976; 11: 27–31.

31. Lam SK: Hypergastrinaemia in cirrhosis of liver. *Gut* 1976; 17: 700–708.

32. Lam SK, Wong H, Ng MMT: Hypersomatostatinaemia in duodenal ulcer. *J Gastroenterol Hepatol* 1986; 1: 119–127.

33. Walsh JH, Lam SK: Gastrin physiology and pathology. In: *Gastrointestinal Hormones. Clinics in Gastroenterology* (ed. Creuts feldt W), WB Saunders, London, Philadelphia and Toronto, 1980; 9: 567–91.

34. Feldman M, Richardson CT, Lam SK, Samloff IM· Comparison of gastric acid secretion rates and serum pepsinogen I and II concentrations in occidental and oriental duodenal ulcer patients. *Gastroenterology* 1988;95: 630–635.

35. Hui WM, Liu HC, Lam SK, Koo A. Histamine containing cells in gastric fundus of dogs. *Cell Mol Biol* 1987; 33: 747–754.

36. Hui WM, Liu HC, Lam SK: Enterochromaffin-like cells of the human stomach — demonstration of histamine content and cholinergic nerve supply. *Cell Mol Biol* 1988;34: 303–309.

37. Ho, J, Lui I, Hui WM, Ng MTT, Lam SK: A study of the correlation of duodenal-ulcer healing with campylobacter-like organisms. *J Gastroenterol Hepatol* 1986; 1: 69–74.

38. Hui WM, Lam SK, Chau PY, Ho J, Lau WY, Poon KP, Lai CL, Lok ASF, Lui IOL, Ng MMT: Pathogenetic role of Campylobacter pyloridis in gastric ulcer. *J Gastroenterol Hepatol* 1987; 2: 309–316.

39. Hui WM, Lam SK, Chau PY, Ho J, Lui I, Lai CL, Lok ASF, Ng MMT: Persistence of Campylobacter pyloridis despite healing of duodenal ulcer and improvement of accompanying duodenitis and gastritis. *Dig Dis Sci* 1987; 32: 1255–1260.

40. Ho J, Hui WM, Ng I, Lam SK: Natural history of Campylobacter pylori in duodenal ulceration treated with an H_2-antagonist. *Aliment Pharmacol Therap* 1989; 3315–3320.

41. Koo J, Ngan YK, Lam SK: Trends in hospital admission, perforation and mortality of peptic ulcer in Hong Kong from 1970–1980. *Gastroenterology* 1982; 84: 1558–1562.

42. Lam SK, Piper DW: Geographical variations in peptic ulcer. *J Gastroenterol Hepatol* 1988; 3: 399–401.

43. Lam SK, Piper DW, Byth K, Ng MMT, Hui WM, McKintosh J. Peptic ulcer rates and trends in Hong Kong and Sydney — A tale of two cities. *J Gastroenterol Hepatol* 1988; 3 (Suppl 1): 16.

44. Lam SK, Hui WM, Ng MMT: Relationship of perforated peptic ulcer to socio-economic stress over the past 26 years in Hong Kong. *Gastroenterological Society of Australia Annual Scientific Meet ing, Alice Springs, 1987;* p. 23.

45. Hui WM, Lam SK. Monthly variation in duodenal ulcer frequency and maximal acid output. *J Gastroenterol Hepatol* 1988; 3: 457–463.

46. Lam SK, Koo J. New approach with old medicine: antacids and bismuth. In: *Drugs and Peptic Ulcer* (ed. Pfeiffer CJ), Uniscience Series on Gastrointestinal Disease, CRC Press, Inc., U.S.A., 1982; 1. 159–182.

47. Lam SK: Antacids: past, present and future. In: *Peptic Ulcer. Clinics in Gastroenterology* (ed. DW Piper), WB Saunders, London, Philadelphia, Torronto, 1988; 2: 641–654.

48. Halter F, Lam SK: Action of antacids: more than bulk neutralization? In: *Advances in Drug Therapy of Gastrointestinal Ulceration* (ed. Garner A), John Wiley & Sons, Chichester, 1989 (in press).

49. Halter F, Lam SK: Antacid therapy and ulcer disease. In: *Ulcer Disease: Investigation and Basis for Therapy* (eds. Swabb EA, Szabo S), 1990 (in press).

50. Lam SK, Lai CL, Lee LNW, Fok KH, Ng MMT, Siu KF: Factors influencing healing of duodenal ulcer. Control of nocturnal secretion by H_2 blockade and characteristics of patients who failed to heal. *Dig Dis Sci* 1985; 30: 45–51.

51. Lam SK, Lai CL, Ng MMT, Fok KH, Hui WM: Duodenal ulcer healing by separate reduction of postprandial and nocturnal secretions have different pathophysiology. *Gut* 1985; 26: 1038–1044.

52. Lam SK: Update on management of peptic ucler. *Med Progress* 1986; 27–34.

53. Lam SK, Hui WM, Ng MMT, Lok ASF, Lai CL, Branicki F, Lau WY, Poon GP: Reducing meal-stimulated acid secretion versus reducing nocturnal acid secretion for the healing of duodenal ulcer. *Dig Dis Sci* 1989 (in press).

54. Hui WM, Liu HC, Lam SK: Parietal cells in duodenal ulcer dis ease: a histochemical study of the effects of omeprazole and ranitidine on mitochondrial activities. *J Gastroenterol Hepatol* 1989;4: 143–149.

55. Hui WM, Lam SK, Lau WY, Branicki FJ, Lok ASF, Ng MMT, Lai CL, Poon GP: Omeprazole and ranitidine in duodenal ulcer healing and subsequent relapse — A randomized double-bllind study with weekly endoscopic assessment. *J Gastroenterol Hepatol* 1989 (in press).

56. Lam SK, Sung JL, Choi: Omeprazole, the first proton pump inhibitor. *J Gastroenterol Hepatol* 1989 (in press).

57. Koo J, Lam SK, Smaje LH: *Microcirculation of the Alimentary Tract*, World Scientific Publishing Co. Pte. Ltd., Singapore, 1983.

58. Hui WM, Lam SK, Ho J, Ng MTT, Lui I, Lai CL, Lok A, Lau WY, Poon GP, Choi S, Choi TK: Chronic antral gastritis in duodenal ucler — Natural history and treatment with prostaglandin E. *Gastroenterology* 1986; 91: 1095–1101.

59. Lam SK, Lau WY, Choi TK, Lai CL, Lok ASF, Hui WM, Ng MMT, Choi SKY: Prostaglandin E1 (misoprostol) overcomes the adverse effect of chronic cigarette smoking on duodenal-ulcer healing. *Dig Dis Sci* 1986; 31: 68S–74S.

60. Lam SK: Peptic ulcer — Medical management. *Abstracts 8th Asian-Pacific Congress of Gastroenterology* 1988; p. 34.

61. Lam SK: Use of cytoprotective agents in the treatment of gastric ulcers. *Med J Aust* 1985; 142: S21–23.

62. Lam SK: Unique advantages of prostaglandin E analogues in peptic ulcer diseases. In: *Prostaglandins in the Upper Gastrointestinal Tract*, Therapeutics Today Series. ADIS Press, Australia, 1986; 5: 26–33.

63. Lam SK: Cytoprotective agents in gastric disorders. *World Therap Dig* 1986; 1: 2–4.

64. Lam SK: Cytoprotective agents come of age. *World Therap Dig* 1986; 1: 2–4.

65. Lam SK: Prostaglandins for duodenal ulcer. *Clin Invest Med* 1987; 10: 232–237.

66. Lam SK: Prostaglandins for duodenal ulcer and gastric ulcer. *J Gastroenterol Hepatol* 1986; 1: 471–481.

67. Koo J, Ho J, Lam SK, Ong GB: Selective coating of gastric ulcer by tripotassium dicitrato bismuthate in the rat. *Gastroenterology* 1982; 82: 864–870.

68. Koo J, Lam SK, Ong GB: Recurrent ulcer treated with colloidal bismuth. *Med J Aust* 1983; 1: 103–104.

69. Koo J, Lam SK: Discriminant factors of gastric ulcer healing by colloidal bismuth. *J Gastroenterol Hepatol* 1987; 2: 473–483.

70. Koo J, Ho JCI, Lam SK, Wong J, Ong GB: Colloidal bismuth in the treatment of experimental gastric ulcer: mechanism of action, 1: Histochemical study. In: Umehara S, Ito H, eds.

71. Lam SK, Misiewicz JJ, Aarimaa M: Site protection and cytoprotection in the management of peptic ulcer and oesophagitis. *Scand J Gastroenterol* 1987; 22 (Suppl 140): 1–64.

72. Sabesin SM, Lam SK: International Sucralfate Research Conference. *Am J Med* 1987; 83 (Suppl 3B): 1–127.

73. Chen BW, Hui WM, Lam SK, Cho CH, Ng MMT, Luk CT: Effect of sucralfate on gastric mucosal blood flow in rats. *Gut* 1989

(in press).

74. Lam SK, Sabesin SM: Acid, cytoprotection, and peptic ulcer. *Am J Med* 1987; 83(3B): 1–3.
75. Hui WM, Lam SK, Ho J, Ng I, Lau WY, Branicki FJ, Lai CL, Lok ASF, Ng MMT, Fok PJ, Poon GP, Choi TK: The effect of sucralfate and cimetidine on duodenal ulcer associated antral gastritis and campylobacter pylori. *Am J Med* 1989 (in press).
76. Lam SK, Hui WM, Lam WY, Branicki FJ, Lai CL, Lok ASF, Ng MTT, Fok PJ, Poon GP, Choi TK: Sucralfate overcomes adverse effect of cigarette smoking on duodenal ulcer healing and prolongs subsequent remission. *Gastroenterology* 1987; 92: 1193–1201.
77. Lam SK, Lau WY, Lai CL, Lee NW, Poon GP, Hui WM, Lok A, Ng MMT, Fok KH, Yu HC: Efficacy of sucralfate in corpus, prepyloric, and duodenal-ulcer associated gastric ulcers. A double-blind, placebo-controlled study. *Am J Med* 1985; 79(2C): 24–31.
78. Lam SK, Koo J: Accurate prediction of duodenal-ulcer healing rate by discriminant analysis. *Gastroenterology* 1983; 85: 403-13-12.
79. Lam SK: The stomach. In: *Current Gastroenterology* (ed. Gitnick GL,), Year Book Medical Publishers, Chicago, London, 1986; pp. 33–62.
80. Lam SK: How does sucralfate heal ulcers? In: Sucralfate; the truth of the story (ed. Tytgat GNJ). *Scand J Gastroenterol* 1989 (in press).
81. Lam SK, Lee NW, Koo J, Hui WM, Fok KH, Ng M: A randomized cross-over trial of tripotassium dicitrato bismuthate versus high dose cimetidine for duodenal ulcers resistant to standard dose of cimetidine. *Gut*, 1984; 25: 703–706.
82. Domschke W, Lam SK, Pounder RE, Andersen D: H_2-Blocker-resistant duodenal ulceration. *Gastroenterol International* 1989; 2: 85–91.
83. Lam SK: Implications of sucralfate induced ulcer healing and relapse. *Am J Med* 1989 (in press).
84. Lam SK: Perspectives of medical treatment for peptic ulcer. In: *Ulcer Disease: Investigation and Basis for Therapy* (ed. Swabb EA, Szabo S), 1989 (in press).
85. Koo J, Lam SK, Chan P, Lee NW, Lam P, Wong J, Ong GB: Proximal gastric vagotomy, truncal vagotomy and drainage, and truncal vagotomy and antrectomy for chronic duodenal ulcer. A prospective, randomized controlled trial. *Ann Surg* 1983; 197: 265–271.
86. Koo J, Lam SK, Ong GB: Cimetidine versus surgery for recurrent ulcer after gastric surgery. *Ann Surg* 1982; 195: 406–412.
87. Lam SK, Chan PKW, Wong J, Ong GB: Fasting and postprandial gastrin before and after highly selective vagotomy, truncal vagotomy and pyloroplasty and truncal vagotomy with antrectomy — Is there a cholinergic antral gastrin inhibitory and releasing mechanism? *Brit J Surg* 1978; 65: 797–800.
88. Koo J, Lam SK: Individual prediction of ulcer recurrence after vagotomy for chronic duodenal ulcer by discriminant analysis. *Gastroenterology* 1983; 85: 413–419.
89. Koo J, Lam SK, Boey J, Lee NW: Gastric acid secretion and its predictive value after vagotomy for perforated duodenal ucler. *Scand J Gastroenterol* 1983; 18: 929–934.
90. Hui WM, Ng MMT, Lok ASF, Lam SK, Yau HH, Lau YN, Lai CL: A randomized prospective study of the efficacy of LASER, heater probe and bipolar electrocoagulation in active bleeding ulcers. *Gastroenterology* 1989; 96: A222.
91. Petersen GM, Lam SK, Samloff IM, Jing L, Rotter JI: Peptic ulcer disease: ulcer therapy as a gene-environment interaction. *Gastroenterolog*, 1989 (in press).
92. Hui WM, Lam SK, Ng MMT, Lai CL, Lok ASF: Long term maintenance therapy for duodenal ulcer: a comparison of 8 forms of treatments. *Gastroenterology* 1989; 96: A222.
93. Koo J, Lam SK, Koo A: The antagonistic effects of vagotomy, pirenzapine and cimetidine on the acetylcholine-, histamine- and gastrin-receptors in the vascular smooth muscle of the rat gas tric microcirculation. In: *Microcirculation of the Alimentary Tract* (eds. Koo A, Lam SK, Smaje), World Scientific Publishing Co. Pte. Ltd., Singapore, 1983; pp. 327–338.

94.   Hui WM, Ho J, Chen BW, Cho CH, Lam SK: The effect of sucralfate on vascular injury and its relation to gastric macroscopic and microscopic mucosal damage induced by ethanol. *Gastroenterology* 1989; 96: A222.

95.   Cho CH, Chen BW, Poon YK, Ng MMT, Hui WM, Lam SK, Ogle CW: Dual effects of zinc sulphate on ethanol-induced injury in rats: possibly mediated by an action on mucosal blood flow. *Dig Dis & Sci* 1989 (in press).

96.   Murakami M, Lam SK, Inada M, Miyake T: Pathophysiology and pathogenesis of acute gastric mucosal lesions following hypother-mic restraint stress in rats. *Gastroenterology* 1985; 88: 660–665.

97.   Chen BW, Hui WM, Lam SK, Ng MMT, Cho CH, Luk CT: Effect of misoprostol and omeprazole on gastric mucosal blood flow in rats — A comparative study by laser-doppler flowmetry. *J Gastroenterol Hepatol* 1988; 3 (Suppl 1): 14.

98.   Hui WM, Chen BW, Cho CH, Lam SK, Luk CT: The effect of components of sucralfate on gastric mucosal blood flow — Does antacid increase mucosal blood flow? *Gastroenterology* 1989; 96: A221.

99.   Hui WM, Lam SK: Etiology and management of chronic gastritis. *Digestive Diseases* 1989; 7: 51–60.

100. Hui WM, Lam SK, Ho J, Lui I, Lau WY, Branicki FJ, Lai CL, Lok ASF, Ng MMT. Omeprazole improves antral gastritis associated with duodenal ulcer (DU). *Gut* 1987; 28: A1340.

101. Hui WM, Lam SK, Lok ASF, Ng MTT, Wong KL, Fok KH: Sulpiride imporves functional dyspepsia — A double blind controlled study. *J Gastroenterol Hepatol* 1986; 1: 391–399.

102. Lam SK, Wong KP, Chan PKW, Ngan H, Ong GB: Recurrent pyogenic cholangitis: a study by endoscopic retrograde cholangiography. *Gastroenterology*, 1978; 74: 1196–1203.

103. Chan CW, Lam SK: Diseases caused by liver flukes and cholangio-carcinoma. In: Tropical Gastroenterology. Bailliere's Clinical Gastroenterology (ed. Gyr KE), Bailliere Tindall, London, Philadelphia, Toronto, Sydney, Tokyo, 1987; 1: 297–318.

104. Lam SK: A study of endoscopic sphincterotomy in recurrent pyogenic cholangitis. *Brit J Surg* 1984; 71: 262–266.

105. Lam SK, Chan CW: Diseases of the biliary tract and the gall bladder. In: *Tropical Gastroenterology. Clinics in Gastroenterology* (ed. Gyr K), WB Saunders, London, Philadelphia, Torronto, 1987; 1: 297–318.

S.K. LAM and W.M. HUI

Research in Hepatology I

Hepatology began as a part of the gastroenterology division, but in recent years, the Department of Medicine has caught up with the rest of the world and given Hepatology its due recognition as a distinct specialty. The Hepatology team now consists of Dr. CL Lai, reader; Dr. Anna SF Lok, senior lecturer and Dr. HT Chung, medical officer.

Apart from the traditional weekly combined GI/liver clinic at Sai Ying Pun, a Hepatitis Clinic was established in Queen Mary Hospital in 1984. In addition, there are separate clinics for patients in various clinical studies.

The birth of Hepatology as a new specialty in the Department led to the creation of a Hepatology Research Fund in 1984. Most of the funding came from pharmaceutical companies in support of clinical studies. Separate funding for laboratory based research came from the University and Strategic Research Grant Committee.

The Hepatology team's research has been focused on hepatitis B and hepatocellular carcinoma — the most prevalent liver diseases in Hong Kong. Hepatitis serology assays were initially performed within the Department. With increasing demand for such assays and the availability of commercial test kits, routine hepatitis serology assays are currently performed by the Virus Unit, Queen Mary Hospital. The Hepatology team has devoted its attention to the development of more sophisticated molecular virologic techniques such as: micromethod for the assay of DNA polymerase (1), tests for hepatitis B virus (HBV) DNA in serum by spot hybridization and lately polymerase chain reaction, using plasma derived, cloned and oligonucleotide HBV probes (2–4), analysis of HBV DNA and HBV RNA in liver and other tissues by Southern and Northern blot hybridization (5) and in vitro evaluation of antiviral agents using transfected cell lines. In 1987, a part of the Department's general laboratory was designated for biohazard work.

The Department's research on hepatitis B dated back to 1975 when Lee first demonstrated a high prevalence of hepatitis B antigen in local patients with chronic liver diseases (6). This was later confirmed by Lam *et al* who showed that HBV infection was the most important cause of liver cirrhosis in Hong Kong Chinese (7). Lee *et al* went on to show that in Chinese populations, hepatitis B infection was frequently transmitted from maternal carriers (8). Lok *et al* confirmed the importance of transmission from maternal carriers as well as intrafamilial spread from carrier fathers or siblings (9). The endemicity of hepatitis B infection in Hong Kong with 50% of the population being infected before reaching adult life may in part contribute to the absence of transmission of hepatitis B by fibreoptic upper gastrointestinal endoscopy (10).

With the availability of hepatitis B vaccines, the Hepatology team played an important role in evaluating these vaccines prior to their general use (11–13). The strategy for screening prior to vaccination was examined (14). The response to hepatitis B vaccine in family members of hepatitis B carriers was studied (15) and the need for vaccination in subjects with isolated antibody to hepatitis B core antigen evaluated (14, 16).

Careful follow-up of a large cohort of patients with chronic HBV infection revealed that the natural history of chronic HBV infection in Chinese patients is very different from that in Caucasians (17–21). The volume of data generated from our studies has convinced investigators world-wide that the patterns of hepatitis B are different in different places (18). Carrier children were usually highly viremic but had minimal liver disease (19). The level of HBV replication generally decreased with age and duration of infection (3). The transition from replicative to non-replicative phase of HBV infection was rapid and smooth in some patients but protracted and fluctuating in others (20). In the latter patients, fluctuations in level of HBV replication were often associated with recurrent exacerbations which may be mistaken for acute hepatitis B (21). These exacerbations were more often seen in patients who received cytotoxic therapy and may precipitate fatal hepatic failure (22).

The Hepatology team has a long-standing commitment in the therapy of HBV infection. In 1978, Lam *et al* published their study on the effect of isoprinosine in acute viral hepatitis (23). This was followed by two reports on the deleterious effect of prednisone in HBV-related chronic active hepatitis (24, 25). The study on prednisone remains the only randomized controlled trial of steriod in chronic hepatitis B and is widely quoted. As of 1984, the Hepatology team has been playing a leading role in the evaluation of antiviral therapy in chronic HBV infection (26–28). The team reported the world's largest, unicentre randomized controlled trial of alpha-interferon in the treatment of chronic hepatitis B (29) and is one of the few centres in the world to have conducted randomized controlled trials of interferon in carrier children (30). Although our initial results were disappointing, i. e. the response to interferon therapy being lower in Chinese compared to Caucasian patients, our current trials are more encouraging. Prednisone priming appears to have a marginal improvement on the antiviral response in carrier children (31) while 50% of adults with elevated transaminase levels have sustained suppression of HBV replication after interferon treatment (32).

In view of the strong association between chronic HBV infection and hepatocellular carcinoma (HCC), the Hepatology team conducted studies to identify factors that determine the development of HCC in hepatitis B carriers (33) and to evaluate the role of alpha-fetoprotein monitoring in the detection of early HCC (34). In addition, the team also performed molecular hybridization studies in serum and liver tissues from patients with HCC for the detection of free and integrated HBV DNA (5, 35, 36).

In the last 15 years, the Department of Medicine, under the guidance of Professor Todd, witnessed the birth of a new specialty which has grown rapidly and achieved international recognition. There is no doubt that the Hepatology team will continue to maintain its high commitment to providing good medical care to patients, to promoting the teaching of Hepatology to students and trainee physicians and to excel in research.

References

1.   Lin HJ, Wu PC, Lai CL and Chak W: Phosphonoformate inhibition assay of hepatitis B viral DNA polymerase: a micromethod. *Clin Biochem* 1984; 30: 549–552.

2.   Lin HJ, Wu PC, Lai CL and Leong S: Molecular hybridization study of plasma hepatitis B virus DNA from different carriers. *J Infect Dis* 1986; 154: 983–989.

3.   Lok ASF, Lai CL, Wu PC, Leung EKY, Lam TS: Spontaneous hepatitis B e antigen to antibody seroconversion and reversion in Chinese patients with chronic hepatitis B virus infection. *Gastroenterology* 1987; 92: 1839–43.

4.   Lin HJ, Wu PC and Lai CL: An oligonucleotide probe for detection of hepatitis B virus DNA in serum. *J Virol Methods* 1987; 15: 139–149.

5.   Lok ASF, Ma OCK: Persistent hepatitis B virus (HBV) replication in Chinese patients with hepatocellular carcinoma (HCC). *Hepatology* 1988; 8: 1431.

6.   Lee AKY: Hepatitis B antigen and auto-antibodies in chronic liver diseases in Hong Kong. *Aust NZ J Med* 1975; 5: 235–239.

7.   Lam KC, Lai CL, Wu PC, Todd D: Etiological spectrum of liver cirrhosis in the Chinese. *J Chron Dis* 1980; 33: 375–381.

8.   Lee AKY, Ip HMH, Wong VCW: Mechanisms of maternal-fetal transmission of hepatitis B virus. *J Infect Dis* 1978; 138: 668–71.

9.   Lok ASF, Lai CL, Wu PC, Wong VCW, Yeoh EK, Lin HJ: Hepatitis B virus infection in Chinese families in Hong Kong. *Am J Epidemiol* 1987; 126: 492–499.

10.   Lok ASF, Lai CL, Hui WM, Ng MMT, Wu PC, Lam SK, Leung EKY: Absence of transmission of hepatitis B by fibreoptic upper gastrointestinal endoscopy. *J Gastroenterol Hepatol* 1987; 2: 175–180.

11.   Lai CL, Wu PC, Lin HJ: Comparison of two hepatitis B vaccines: preliminary report of a randomized trial. In: *Viral Hepatitis B Infection in the Western Pacific Region: Vaccine and Control* (eds. Lam SK, Lai CL, Yoeh EK), World Scientific Publishing Co., Singapore, 1984; pp. 199–209.

12.   Lai CL, Yeoh EK, Chang WK, Lo VWL, Ng LNK: Use of the hepatitis B recombinant DNA yeast vaccine (H-B-VAX II) in children: two doses vs. three doses of 5 ug regime; an interim report. *J Infect* 1986; 13 (Suppl): 19–25.

13.   Lau JYN, Lai CL, Wu PC, Lin HJ: Comparison of two plasma-derived hepatitis B vac-

cines: long-term report of a prospective, randomized trial. *J Gastroenterol Hepatol* 1989; 4: 331–338.

14. Lok ASF, Lai CL, Wu PC: Prevalence of isolated antibody to hepatitis B core antigen in an area endemic for hepatitis B virus infection: implications in hepatitis B vaccination programs. *Hepatology* 1988; 8: 766–770.

15. Lok ASF, Lai CL, Wu PC, Ng MMT: Response to hepatitis B vaccine in family members of HBsAg carriers. *J Med Virol* 1986; 19: 33–39.

16. Lok ASF, Lai CL, Wu PC: Response to hepatitis B vaccine in subjects positive for anti-HBc. In: *Asian Symposium on Strategies for Large Scale Hepatitis B Immunization* (ed. Goulli NE), HK Sci Press, 1988; pp. 141–146.

17. Lam KC, Lai CL, Chan WC: Clinical features and natural mortality of chronic active hepatitis in Hong Kong. *Aust NZ J Med* 1981; 11: 354–358.

18. Lok ASF: Acute viral hepatitis in chronic carriers of hepatitis B virus: different patterns in different places. *Hepatology* 1989; 10: 252–253.

19. Lok ASF, Lai CL: A longitudinal follow-up of asymptomatic hepatitis B surface antigen-positive Chinese children. *Hepatology* 1988; 8: 1130–1133.

20. Lok ASF, Lai CL: Acute exacerbations in Chinese patients with chronic hepatitis B virus infection: incidence, etiology and predisposing factors. *J Hepatol* (in press).

21. Lau JYN, Lai CL, Lin HJ, Lok ASF, Liang RHS, Wu PC, Chan TK, Todd D: Fatal reactivation of chronic hepatitis B virus infection following chemotherapy withdrawal in lymphoma patients. *Q J Med* (in press).

22. Lam KC, Lin HJ, Lai CL, Lam SK, Kwan YL: Isoprinosine in classical acute viral hepatitis. *Am J Dig Dis* 1978; 23: 893–896.

23. Lam KC, Lai CL, Ng RP, Trepo C, Wu PC: Deleterious effect of prednisone in HBsAg-positive chronic active hepatitis. *New England J Med* 1981; 304: 380–386.

24. Wu PC, Lai CL, Lam KC, Ho J: Prednisolone in HBsAg-positive chronic active hepatitis: histologic evaluation in a controlled prospective study. *Hepatology* 1982; 2: 777–783.

25. Lok ASF: Antiviral therapy of chronic hepatitis B virus infection. *J Gastroenterol Hepatol* 1986; 1: 169–179.

26. Lok ASF, Lai CL, Wu PC: Interferon therapy of chronic hepatitis B virus infection in Chinese. *J Hepatol* 1986; 3 (Suppl): S209–S215.

27. Lok ASF: Antiviral therapy of chronic hepatitis B virus infection. In: *Proceedings of the Centennial Conference, Faculty of Medicine, HKU,* 1988; pp. 153–161.

28. Lok ASF, Lai CL, Wu PC, Lau JYN, Leung EKY, Wong LSK: Treatment of chronic hepatitis B with interferon: experience in Asian patients. *Seminars in Liver Diseases* 1989; 9: 249–253.

29. Lok ASF, Lai CL, Wu PC, Leung EKY: Long-term follow-up in a randomized controlled trial of recombinant alpha$_2$-interferon in Chinese patients with chronic hepatitis B infection. *Lancet* 1988; 2: 298–302.

30. Lai CL, Lok SF, Lin HJ, Wu PC, Yeoh EK, Yeung CY: Placebo-controlled trial of recombinant alpha$_2$-interferon in Chinese HBsAg-carrier children. *Lancet* 1987; 2: 877–880.

31. Lai CL, Lok ASF, Lin HJ, Wu PC, Lau JYN and Yeung CY: Use of recombinant alpha$_2$ interferon (r-IFN) with or without steroid in Chinese HBsAg carrier children: a prospective double-blind controlled trial. *Gastroenterology* 1989; 96 (Suppl): A618.

32. Lok ASF, Lai CL, Lau JYN and Wu PC: Effects of age, serum ALT level and prednisone withdrawal on the response to alpha-interferon (IFN) therapy in Chinese patients with chronic HBV infection. *Gastroenterology* 1989; 96 (Suppl): A623.

33. Lok ASF, Lai CL: Factors determining the development of hepatocellular carcinoma in hepatitis B surface antigen carriers: a comparison between families with clusters and solitary cases. *Cancer* 1988; 61: 1287–1291.

34. Lok ASF, Lai CL: Alpha-fetoprotein monitoring in Chinese patients with chronic hepatitis B virus infection: role in the early detection of hepatocellular carcinoma. *Hepatology* 1989; 9: 110–115.

35. Lin HJ, Lai CL, Wu PC: Serum hepatitis B viral DNA in HBsAg-positive hepatocellular carcinoma treated with interferon or adriamycin. *Br J Cancer* 1986; 54: 67–73.

36. Fowler MJF, Greenfield C, Chu CM, Karayiannis P, Dunk A, Lok ASF, Lai CL, Yeoh

EK, Monjardino JP, Wankya BM and Thomas HC: Integration of HBV-DNA may not be a prerequisite for the maintenance of the state of malignant transformation: an analysis of 110 liver biopsies. *J Hepatol* 1986; 2: 218–229.

ANNA S.F. LOK

Hepatocellular Carcinoma (HCC)

HCC is the commonest cancer affecting males in the world and the second commonest cancer in Hong Kong. The probable role of HBV in hepatocarcinogenesis was reviewed in a paper from our Department (1). The evidences were drawn from epidemiological studies, molecular virology and animals infected with the hepadra viruses (a group of viruses phylogenetically related to HBV). In a more recent paper (2), the role of other causative factors, especially cirrhosis and post-transfusion non-A, non-B hepatitis (hepatitis C), were investigated. We concluded that in chronic HBV infection, there was random integration of HBV DNA into the host genome. The cirrhosis associated with HBV infection would enhance HCC development by necroinflammation and increased HBV DNA integration during regeneration of cells. Random HBV DNA integration may trigger the development of malignant clone(s) of cells, leading to HCC.

The clinical features of HCC patients were reviewed in two studies involving 211 and 186 Hong Kong Chinese (3, 4). The male to female ratio was 5 to 1 with a peak incidence of presentation at the sixth decade. The ratio of the serum aspartate aminotransferase (AST) to alanine aminotransferase (ALT) was 1. 4 to 1. AST was produced by mitochondria in hepatocytes. A further study demonstrated that HCC cells showed a higher numerical density and surface density of the internal membrane and cristae of the mitochondria than those of HBsAg-positive cirrhosis (5). This signifies an increased functional activity of mitochondria in HCC.

Only 66% of subjects had an alpha-foetoprotein (AFP) level of over 200 ng/ml. 95% of the subjects were positive for HBsAg in the serum. Males showed a higher proportion with cirrhosis (95%) compared to females (71%) (p = 0. 02). These two findings supports the importance of HBV and cirrhosis in hepatocarcinogenesis (1, 2). Familial clustering of HCC was also described, the reason for the clustering might be genetic and/or environmental (6).

The only two indicators of poor prognosis were a raised bilirubin on presentation (3) and

the presence of clear cells in the hepatocytes (7). Clear cells occur during the intermediary stages in experimental HCC, and may represent an earlier stage of HCC in humans and hence the association with a better prognosis (8). The resectability rate was only 3%. The median survival rate was 3. 5 weeks for untreated patients. Our HCC patients presented late with poor prognosis. Ultrasonographic studies of HCC subjects showed that it was a sensitive and non-invasive method that was almost comparable in accuracy of diagnosis to hepatic arteriogram (9).

Since the majority of our patients has inoperable HCC, the treatment of these patients was therefore systematically studied. Doxorubicin (adriamycin) was the sole agent to be of some proven use in inducing remission. We carried out the first prospective randomized trial of doxorubicin versus no antitumour therapy in the world in 106 patients (10). The median survival rate of the group receiving no antitumour therapy compared with those receiving doxorubicin was improved marginally from 7. 5 weeks to 10. 6 weeks. Doxorubicin induced tumour regression of 25–50% in 5% of subjects and of over 50% in only 3. 3% of subjects. It caused an unacceptable fatal complication rate of 25%. Immunomodulatory agents, specifically recombinant alpha$_2$ interferon, (rIFN) and interleukin 2, were studied. A study randomized 25 subjects on doxorubicin and 50 subjects on two regimes of rIFN, the first prospective randomized trial of rIFN in HCC (11). The survival rate of the subjects receiving either agent was comparable. rIFN was superior to doxorubicin in causing more tumour regression (p = 0. 00199), less progressive tumours (p = 0. 0017) and less severe marrow suppression (p = 0. 01217). The fatal complication due to rIFN (3. 8%) was also less than doxorubicin (25%) (p = 0. 01383). A further study of rIFN vs no antitumour therapy in 71 patients (12) showed an increased median survival from 7. 5 wks to 14 wks (p = 0. 0161). The tumour regression rate associated with rIFN was the same as in the previous study. A parallel study of HBV DNA in subjects treated with rIFN showed that HBV replication could be activated or suppressed in advanced HCC, and that rIFN was effective in suppressing HBV DNA while the patients were being treated (13).

Hepatitis B Vaccination

The ultimate goal for the eradication of HBV associated disease, i. e. , cirrhosis and HCC, is the global eradication of HBV infection by hepatitis B vaccination. Prospective randomized studies were carried out with both the plasma-derived vaccines and the recombinant DNA yeast vaccine.

(A) Plasma-derived vaccines.

A study using the Merck Institute vaccine (HB-VAX) in adults showed that 10 ug dose is as immunogenic, efficacious and safe as the recommended 20 ug dose (14). Another study comparing the vaccine produced by the Institute Pasteur (HEVAC B) and by the Green Cross Corporation, Osaka (GCC VAC) showed that both had comparable immunogenicity and safety, though GCC VAC gave significantly lower but still 'protective' anti-HBs levels (15, 16).

(B) Recombinant DNA yeast vaccines.

This is the first vaccine to be produced by recombinant DNA technology. In a prospective trial in 306 children aged 3 mos to ll years of age, the recipients were randomized to receive (a) 3 doses of HB-VAX, (b) 2 doses of the recombinant vaccine by the Merck Institute (AB-VAX II) or (c) 3 doses of HB-VAX II (17). This study showed that HB-VAX II was comparable to HB-VAX in immunogenicity (98–100%), efficacy and safety. Further, though there was no rise of anti-HBs titres associated with the third dose of HB-VAX II, those receiving only two doses had a geometric mean level of anti-HBs comparable to those receiving three doses on long term follow-up of the vaccines for up to 4 years.

The last 15 years witnessed an explosion of information concerning HCC and the prevention of hepatitis B infection by vaccination. The Department of Medicine has contributed significantly to these fields and has gained recognition in the world for its contributions.

References

1. Lai CL, Wu PC, Yeoh EK, Lok ASF, Lin HJ, Lam SK & Todd D: Hepatocellular carcinoma and the hepatitis B virus. In: *Viral Hepatitis B Infection in the Western Pacific Region: Vaccine and Control*, World Scientific Publications Co., Singapore, 1984; pp. 3–16.
2. Lau JYN & Lai CL: Hepatocarcinogenesis. *Tropical Gastroenterology* (in press).
3. Lai CL, Lam KC, Wong KP, Wu PC & Todd D: Clinical features of hepatocellular carcinoma: review of 211 patients in Hong Kong. *Cancer* 1981; 47: 2746–2755.
4. Lai CL, Gregory PB, Wu PC, Lok ASF, Wong KP & Ng MMT: Hepatocellular carcinoma in Chinese males and females: possible causes for the male predominance. *Cancer* 1987; 60: 1107–1110.
5. Wu PC, Lai CL & Liddell RHA: Quantitative morphology of mitochondria in hepatocellular carcinoma and chronic liver disease. *Arch Path Lab Med* 1984; 108: 914–916.
6. Lok A & Lai CL: Factors determining the development of hepatocellular carcinoma (HCC) in hepatitis B surface antigen carriers: a comparison between families with clusters and solitary cases of hepatocellular carcinoma. *Cancer* 1988; 61: 1287–1291.
7. Lai CL, Wu PC, Lam KC & Todd: Histologic prognostic indicators in hepatocellular carcinoma. *Cancer* 1979; 44: 1677–1680.
8. Wu PC, Lai CL, Lam KC, Lok ASF & Lin HJ: Clear cell carcinoma of liver: an ultrastructural study. *Cancer* 1983; 2: 504–507.
9. Wong KL, Lai CL, Wu PC, Hui WM, Wong KP & Lok ASF: Ultrasonographic studies in hepatic neoplasms: patterns and comparisons with contrast radiological studies. *Clin Radiol* 1985; 36: 511–516.
10. Lai CL, Wu PC, Chan GCB, Lok ASF & Lin HJ: Adriamycin vs no antitumour therapy in inoperable hepatocellular carcinoma: a prospective randomized trial. *Cancer* 1988: 62: 479–483.
11. Lai CL, Wu PC, Lok ASF, Lin HJ, Ngan H, Lau JYN, Chung HT, Ng MMT, Yeoh EK, Arnold M: Recombinant Alpha$_2$ Interferon is superior to Doxorubicin for inoperable hepatocellular carcinoma: a prospective ran-

domized trial. *Br J Cancer* 1989 (in press).

12. Lai CL, Lok ASF, Lau JYN, Wu PC, Lin HJ: A prospective randomized trial of recombinant Alpha$_2$ Interferon (αIFN) vs no anti-tumour treatment in inoperable hepatocellular carcinoma (HCC). *Hepatology* 1988; 8: 1440.

13. Lin HJ, Lai CL & Wu PC: Serum hepatitis B viral DNA in HBsAg-positive hepatocellular carcinoma treated with Interferon or Adriamycin. *Br J Cancer* 1986; 54: 67–73.

14. Yeoh EK, Lai CL, Chang WK & Lo HY: Comparison of the immunogenicity, efficacy and safety of 10 ug and 20 ug of a hepatitis B vaccine: a prospective randomized trial. *J Hyg* 1986; 96: 491–499.

15. Lai CL, Wu PC & Lin HJ: Comparison of two hepatitis B vaccines: preliminary report of a randomized trial. In: *Viral Hepatitis B Infection in the Western Pacific Region: Vaccine and Control* (eds. Lai CL, Lam SK, Yeoh EK), World Scientific Publications Co., Singapore, 1984; pp. 199–209.

16. Lau JYN, Lai CL, Wu PC & Lin HJ: Comparison of two plasma-derived hepatitis B vaccines — Long term report of a prospective trial. *J Gastroenterol & Hepatol* 1989; 4: 331–337.

17. Lai CL, Yeoh EK, Chang WK, Lo V & Ng L: Use of the hepatitis B recombinant DNA yeast vaccine (H-B-VAX II) in children: two doses vs three doses of 5 ug Regime. An interim report. *J Infect* 1986; 13 (Suppl A): 19–25.

C.L. LAI

ACHIEVEMENTS IN HAEMATOLOGY/ONCOLOGY

Haematology as a subspecialty of Medicine has emerged from a difficult period triumphantly due to the leadership of Professor Todd. While in United Kingdom, haematology moved towards being a strong laboratory discipline with only a moderate amount of clinical commitments; here in Hong Kong, we remained an important and distinct division in Medicine and Laboratory Haematology was allowed to develop fully in Pathology. Although amalgamation of the two activities into a Department of Haematology could be possible, it would have been detrimental to both Departments concerned. As it is, the two divisions in Haematology collaborated fully. While almost all special haematology tests were done in Medicine at the beginning of this period, we are now only responsible for cytogenetics of haemic malignancy and radionuclides in diagnostic haematology. This change has allowed us to channel resources to research and development work and accounted for our success during this period. Furthermore, with the work load of a clinician haematologist shifted largely to management of haemic malignancy and bone marrow transplantation, Haematology/Oncology should best be entrenched in Medicine and there will be less pressure for us to change in the future.

Staff: All teaching staff and most rotation registrars have general medical as well as haematology/oncology service duties. Professor D Todd continued to contribute to clinical service and research despite heavy administrative commitments as Head of Department. Other medical staff are: Professor T.K. Chan, Professor S.C. Tso (resigned in 1985), Dr. Ronald Ng (moved to Singapore in 1983), Dr. Raymond H.S. Liang (since 1985), and Dr. Edmond K.W. Chiu (since 1988). We were assisted by rotation registrars as well as elective trainees from paediatrics, gynaecology and radiotherapy. Dr. Vivian Chan, the only biochemist in the Department, moved from Endocrinology to Haematology; initially because of the application of radioimmunoassay to coagulation factors and work on cell culture. Later, she established the DNA laboratory and applied recombinant DNA technology to the study of thalassaemias, haemophilias and haemic malignancy. This has given a great boost to research activities of the haematology team.

Clinical Services: Haematology/Oncology services have expanded to three outpatient sessions (Lymphoma, Leukaemia and Blood), three chemotherapy clinics and one special blood clinic (for Haemophiliacs and Cooley's anaemia) per week. Plasmapheresis and cell pheresis started by Dr. Ronald Ng became more organized in 1985 with a special nurse in the A2 side room and Dr. K.L. Wong, our immunologist, has been mainly in charge of the 150 to 200 pheresis per annum. The haematology team supervises those patients requiring the procedure for hyperviscosity and leucostasis.

Blood cases are accommodated in general medical wards and managed by the general ward clinical staff, we are required to provide regular attendance and consultation for 20 to 40 inpatients, mostly with acute leukamia or lymphoma. Some facilities for isolation of the neutropenic patients was introduced in partitioned cubicles in Wards A2 and E2. A proper reverse isolation unit with 11 rooms in J block extension of Queen Mary Hospital will be available in January, 1990 and bone marrow transplantation will then be performed in Hong Kong.

T.K. CHAN

Research in Haematology

Professor David Todd's inaugural lecture 'Genes, Beans & Marco Polo' depicts two of the main areas of research in Haematology. This centres on the two most common genetic disorders in this part of the world, namely, glucose-6-phosphate dehydrogenase (G6PD) deficiency and thalassemia.

G6PD Deficiency

G6PD deficiency is an X-linked inherited condition which affects 4.66% of the Chinese adult males in Hong Kong. Of the three common variants found here, G6PD Hong Kong-Pokfulam and G6PD B (–) Chinese are two novel variants isolated and characterized by Chan & Todd (1). In the steady state, G6PD deficient subjects were not anaemic and autologous red cell survival in the three common variants were only moderately shortened (2). However, since acute intravascular haemolysis was often noted in G6PD subjects with viral hepatitis, typhoid fever and various illnesses, extensive studies on the haemolytic effects of drugs and illness were made using cross-transfusion of ^{51}Cr-labelled G6PD deficient erythrocytes in normal subjects and autologous survival in G6PD deficient individuals (2, 3, 4). It was concluded that the additional oxidant injury of drugs taken during the illness probably play a causative role in the severe haemolytic episode. A hallmark of oxidative injury 'the erythrocyte hemighost' was associated with acute massive haemolysis in G6PD deficient subjects (5). This cell had damage to its membrane as well as haemoglobin and caused marked sludging in the microcirculation, resulting in renal shutdown and death. Exchange transfusion and forced alkaline diuresis were proposed as the rational treatment and proved successful in a number of patients, including three Pakistani Muslim who succumbed to haemolysis after taking aniline-dyed rice at the post Ramadan feast (6). Finally, although xylitol was suggested as an alternate substrate for the generation of NADPH, Chan & Todd demonstrated that it was ineffective in vitro and failed to protect against primaquine-induced haemolysis in vivo (6, 7).

Thalassemia

1974 saw the advent of the application of DNA technology to haematology with methods of preparing globin mRNA and liquid hybridization. Kan, Todd and co-workers were the first to show that a congenital defect, i. e. homozygous α thalassemia 1 (hydrops fetalis) was due to α gene deletion (8, 9) with concomitant absent of the α globin mRNA (10). The molecular lesions of the α thalassemia syndromes were also characterized (11, 12). This was followed by a series of 'first' discoveries and achievements, the most significant of which was the introduction of prenatal diagnosis for homozygous α thalassemia in 1978. This was the first successful attempt at antenatal diagnosis of a congenital defect (13), which remains todate, the only means of control for these disorders. Other early work included the discovery of the first non-deletion α thalassemia, due to Hb Quong-Sze (14) (named after the birth place of patient), and that HbQ$^{\alpha74\,Asp\text{-}His}$ is always associated with a leftward deletion of the α gene (15, 16). Measurement of Hb Bart's level in umbilical cord blood was used to determine the incidence of α thalassemia (17). However, it was concluded that Hb Bart's level cannot distinguish between α thalassemia 2 and α thalassemia 1 (18), thus there was the need to establish gene mapping technique for this purpose. In 1982, with the help of Prof. Y. W. Kan of the University of California School of Medicine, San Francisco, we set up the DNA laboratory of the Department. We were in fact the first centre in SE Asia to offer prenatal diagnosis of α thalassemia by DNA technology. In addition, improvement was made on the methodology such that diagnosis can be made directly on uncultured amniotic fluid fetal cells (19, 20). We also described the first case of HbH hydrops fetalis due to inheritance of ζ-α thalassemia 1 and non-deletion α thalassemia (21). A method for the prenatal diagnosis of this condition was subsequently derived and successfully applied, based on a restriction fragment length polymorphism (RFLP) in the interzeta hypervariable region (22). A survey of 100 normal non-thalassemic subjects, 110 β thalassemia minor and 47 β thalassemia major patients revealed an α thal-1 incidence of 2.2% and α thal-2 of 1. 8% in the local population (23). This was of value in predicting the workload of the prenatal diagnosis service, aside from rendering insight into the possible ameliorating effect of the coinheritance of α and β thalassemias. However, it was of particular interest to note that one patient with HbH disease and Hb New York had severe anaemia (3.4 –6.9 g/dl) since early childhood, requiring frequent blood transfusion. It appeared that unlike most β variants, β^{NY} has a higher affinity for α^A chain. Thus the preferential formation of Hb New York, which is unstable, would worsen the deficiency of α^A chain already present, accounting for her marked anaemia (24). This is an important observation in view of the common occurrence of Hb New York in South China (25–27). The molecular heterogeneity of HbH disease in the Chinese (28–30), the identification of another type of HbH hydrops fetalis (30) and the two molecular organizations responsible for α thalassemia 2 were also reported (31).

Cooley's anemia or β thalassemia major is due to inheritance of two β thalassemia mutations from the parents. This condition is common in the Mediterranean region, South East Asia and South China. With a 6% incidence of β thal minor in Hong Kong (32), the number of pregnancies at risk for β thal major is 288 per annum. Prenatal diagnosis can be achieved by fetal blood sampling, use of RFLP to link the affected gene or direct analysis of specific mutation using allele specific oligonucleotide (ASO) probes. Since it is known that the incidence of RFLP sites varies in different ethnic groups, a study of 47 unrelated β thalassemia major patients and their families was made to characterize their haplotypes (33, 34), followed by determination of their specific mutations using ASO probes (35). This enabled us to institute a comprehensive thalassemia control program and prenatal diagnosis of β thalassemia has been available locally since 1984. With the recent development of polymerase chain reaction (PCR) amplification of DNA, techniques for these diagnoses have been much simplified. Our experience and strategies in prenatal testing of thalassemias have been extensively reviewed (20, 36–40). Using PCR amplification and direct genomic sequencing, two novel β thalassemia mutations were characterized, these were Codon 14/15 (+G) (41) and Codon 71 (+T) (42), both frameshift mutations resulting in β^0 thalassemia. Fortunately, although at least 11 β thalassemia mutations have been found in the Chinese, the four common variants would account for 90% of cases. We have recently introduced the use of horse-radish peroxidase (HRP) linked ASO probes for direct analysis of these mutations on PCR-amplied genomic DNA (39). This obviates the use of radioisotope and provides a result within 3–4 days of amniocentesis or chorionic villus sampling (CVS).

Other contributions in the area of thalassemia includes clinical observations such as paraparesis with HbE-β thalassemia (43); significance of subnormal red cell folate in thalassemia (44); folate studies in thalassemia (45), splenomegaly in HbH disease (46) and iron overload in thalassemic patients (47, 48) as well as concepts in molecular pathology (49) and management of this disorder (50).

Coagulation and Haemostasis

This forms our third interest in Haematology and began with the identification and localization of Antithrombin III (AtIII), in human tissues (51) using a polyclonal antibody raised here. With the development of a radioimmunoassay for AtIII, it was possible not only to measure serum levels in various disease states with accuracy (52), but one was able to demonstrate that this major natural anticoagulant was synthesised and secreted from the vascular endothelium (53). Both the anti-Xa and thrombin-neutralizing activities of the EC-AtIII were rapid and active even in the absence of added heparin. It was concluded that the major portion was probably bound to endogenous heparin-like substances, thus accounting for its decreased exogenous heparin binding (54). The presence of AtIII and other antithrombic factors in the vascular endothelium offer protection against thrombosis and possibly atherosclerosis. Further studies in heparin-AtIII binding by immuno-electrophoresis, indicated a qualitative change in the AtIII molecule within 5 min of heparin injection and throughout heparin therapy as well as a progressive quantitative decrease as a result of increased turnover of AtIII. The qualitative and quantitative changes observed probably accounted for the thrombotic tendency (55) after prolonged heparin infusion. Also serial measurement of AtIII would be a useful prediction of post-operative deep vein thrombosis (DVT) (52). Measurements of changes in plasminogen activator, fibrinogen degradation products and AtIII levels during venous occlusion provided knowledge on the body's antithrombotic mechanisms and reflects an individual's global response to venous stasis (56).

Various clinical studies made in this area included DVT after stroke (57), venous thrombosis in Haemoglobin H disease patients following splenectomy (58) and DVT and changes in coagulation and fibrinolysis after gynaecological operations (59). A comparative study was made on DVT and the effects of oral contraceptives and malignant diseases in Chinese and Caucasian patients (60). It seems that enhanced fibrinolytic activity and absence of a fall in AtIII level post-operatively may explain the lower incidence of DVT in Chinese (59, 60).

While the low AtIII level in diabetic and non-diabetic nephropathy, as a result of urinary loss, contributes to the pathogenesis of intraglomerular thrombosis and deteriorating renal function (61); the low level in cirrhosis and carcinoma of liver reflects increased consumption or catabolism of AtIII rather than decreased production (62). Hypofibrinogenemia due to increased fibrinolysis was associated with acute promyelocytic leukaemia and prompt treatment with tranexamic acid was effective in controlling fatal bleeding (63).

The role of different hypoglycaemic agents on platelet function, fibrinolysis, coagulation and microangiopathy were compared in patients with diabetic retinopathy in a 2 year prospective longitudinal study. Gliclazide was found to be more effective in arresting the progression of diabetic retinopathy (64, 65).

Factor VIII is one of the clotting factors in the coagulation cascade, it circulates in plasma as a complex of two proteins, the VIII related protein (VIII: RAG) or von Willebrand factor (vWF) and the VIII procoagulant (VIII: C). Deficiency of either part will result in either von Willebrand disease or Haemophilia A, the two commonest congenital bleeding disorders in man. Our analysis of Factor VIII: R isolated from cultured human endothelial cells showed that it is synthesised as subunits and assembled into tetramers and higher

multimers before secretion from the cells. Decreased synthesis or defective assembly would result in von Willebrand's Disease (66). Cell-free translation of the VIII: RAG indicated that the VIII: R mRNA is responsible for the synthesis of subunits only and intracellular post-translational events are required for assembly of multimers (67).

Studies on the molecular defect of Haemophilia A started in 1987 with an aim to offer prenatal diagnosis for this disorder. Thirty-one haemophiliac A patients, 130 family members and 23 unrelated normal males were studied to determine the most suitable RFLP sites for linkage with the affected gene. We found that using a combination of four polymorphisms, namely BclI, XbaI, TaqI-St14 systems I & II, it would be possible to offer carrier detection or prenatal diagnosis in 96% of Chinese females at risk (68). More recently, we reported on two additional XbaI sites which could be useful in prenatal diagnosis (69). The prenatal testing and carrier detection service for Haemophilia A has been available since 1987 (70). A screening of all the haemophiliacs with Factor VIII cDNA probe revealed one patient with a novel EcoRI site mutation. This was characterized by selective PCR of exon 4 of the factor VIII gene, followed by direct genomic sequencing. This missense mutation is the first described which affects an EcoRI site and results in moderately severe disease (71).

Studies of the molecular lesions of Haemophila B is currently in progress.

Since 1983, the Department of Medicine and the Department of Obstetrics & Gynaecology, University of Hong Kong, have jointly established the first and only Prenatal Diagnosis Clinic for congenital disorders using DNA technology in Hong Kong. This service is available to all Hong Kong citizens and funded by the Government Hospital Authority.

References

1.   Chan TK, Todd D: Characteristics and distribution of G6PD deficient variants in South China. *Am J Hum Genet* 1972; 24: 475–478.

2.   Chan TK, Todd D, Tso SC: Red cell survival studies in glucose-6-phosphate dehy-

drogenase deficiency. *Bull HK Med Assoc* 1974; 26: 41–48.

3. Chan TK, Todd D: Haemolysis complicating viral hepatitis in patients with glucose-6-phosphate dehydrogenase deficiency. *Br Med J* 1975; 1: 131–133.

4. Chan TK, Todd D, Tso SC: Drug-induced haemolysis in glucose-6-phosphate dehydrogenase deficiency. *Br Med J* 1976; 2: 1227–1229.

5. Chan TK, Chan WC, Weed RI: Erythrocyte hemighosts: a hallmark of severe oxidative injury in vivo. *Br J Haematol* 1982; 50: 575–582.

6. Chan TK: Acute massive intravascular haemolysis in Pakistani after Ramadan. *Proc 5th Meeting Asian Pacific Div, Int Soc Haematol*, Manila, 1983; p. 34.
Chan TK: Glucose-6-phosphate dehydrogenase deficiency. MD thesis, University of Hong Kong, 1983.

7. Chan TK, Todd D: Can xylitol infusion prevent oxidative haemolysis in G6PD deficiency? *Proc 3rd Meeting Eur and Afr Div, Int Soc Haematol*, London, 1975.

8. Taylor JM, Dozy AM, Kan YW, Varmus HE, Lie-Injo LE, Ganesan J, Todd D. Genetic lesion in homozygous alpha-thalassaemia (hydrops foetalis). *Nature* 1974; 251: 392–393.

9. Kan YW, Taylor JM, Dozy AM, Varmus HE, Lie-Injo LE, Ganesan J, Todd D: Homozygous alpha-thalassemia (hydrops fetalis): evidence for deletion of the α structure gene. In: *Erythrocyte Structure and Function*, Alan R Liss Inc, New York, 1975; 1: 139–146.

10. Kan YW, Todd D, Holland JP, Dozy AM: Absence of alpha-globin mRNA in homozygous alpha-thalassaemia. *J Clin Ivest* 1974; 53: 37a.

11. Kan YW, Dozy AM, Varmus HE, Taylor JM, Holland JP, Lie-Injo LE, Ganesan J, Todd D: The molecular basis of the alpha thalassemia syndromes. *Clin Res* 1975; 23: 398.

12. Kan YW, Dozy AM, Varmus HE, Taylor JM, Holland JP, Lie Injo LE, Ganesan J, Todd D: Deletion of alpha-globin genes in haemoglobin-H disease demonstrates multiple alpha globin structural loci. *Nature* 1975; 255: 255–256.

13. Wong V, Ma HK, Todd D, Golbus MS, Dozy AM, Kan YW. Diagnosis of homozygous α-thalassemia in cultured amniotic fluid fibroblasts. *N Engl J Med* 1978; 298: 669–670.

14. Kan YW, Dozy AM, Trecartin R, Todd D: Identification of a non-deletion defect in α-thalassemia. *N Engl J Med* 1977; 297: 1081–1083.

15. Lie-Injo LE, Dozy AM, Kan YW, Lopes M, Todd D: The α-globin gene in the variant HbQ[74 Asp-His]. *Proc 4th Meeting Asian Pacific Div, Int Soc Hematol*, Seoul, 1979; p. 76.

16. Lie-Injo LE, Dozy AM, Kan YW, Lopes M, Todd D: The α-globin gene adjacent to the gene for Hb Q-α[74 His-Asp] is deleted, but not that adjacent to the gene for Hb G-α[30 Glu-Gln]; three fourths of the a globin genes are deleted in Hb Q-α-thalassemia. *Blood* 1979; 54: 1407–1416.

17. Li AMC, Lee FT, Todd D: The screening of Chinese cord blood for haemoglobinopathies. *Human Hered* 1982; 32: 62–70.

18. Todd D, Chan TK: Haemoglobin Bart's levels in umbilical cord blood: failure as a method for distinguishing mild from severe α-thalassemia trait in the Chinese. *Hemoglobin* 1978; 2: 389–392.

19. Chan V, Ghosh A, Chan TK, Wong V, Todd D: Prenatal diagnosis of homozygous α thalassemia by direct DNA analysis of uncultured amniotic fluid cells. *Br Med J* 1984; 288: 1327–1330.

20. Chan V, Chan TK, Todd D: Prenatal diagnosis of homozygous α-thalassemia (Hemoglobin Bart's hydrops fetalis). In: *Prenatal Diagnosis of Thalassemia and the Hemoglobinopathies*. (ed. Loukopoulous D), CRC Press, Florida, 1988; Ch 16, pp. 209–220.

21. Chan V, Chan TK, Liang ST, Ghosh A, Kan YW, Todd D. Hydrops fetalis due to an unusual form of HbH disease. *Blood* 1985; 66: 224–228.

22. Chan V, Chan TK, Wong ACK, Chan TPT, Ghosh A, Todd D. Restriction fragment length polymorphism in the interzeta hypervariable region for prenatal diagnosis of non-deletion α-thalassemia. *Am J Hematol* 1988; 27: 242–246.

23. Chan V, Chan TK, Cheng MY, Kan YW, Todd D: Organization of the ζ-α genes in Chinese. *Br J Haematol* 1986; 64: 97–105.

24. Chan V, Chan TK, Tso SC, Todd D: Combination of three α-globin gene loci deletions

and Hemoglobin New York results in a severe Hemoglobin H syndrome. *Am J Hematol* 1987; 24: 301–306.

25. Todd D, Chan V, Schneider RG, Dozy AM, Kan YW, Chan TK: Globin chain synthesis in haemoglobin New York. *Br J Haematol* 1980; 46: 557–564.

26. Todd D, Chan V, Chan TK: Haemoglobinopathies/thalassemia in Southern Chinese. *The 21st Congress Int Soc Haematol*, Sydney, 1986; Sym M 4–5, p 102.

27. Todd D: Thalassemia and haemoglobinopathies. *Medicine* 1980; 27: 1406–1412.

28. Kan YW, Todd D, Dozy AM: Haemoglobin Constant Spring synthesis in red cell precursors. *Br J Haematol* 1974; 28: 103–108.

29. Todd D: Haemoglobin Constant Spring and human haemoglobin synthesis. *Proc 4th Meeting Asian Pacific Div, Int Soc Haematol,*1979; 253–255.

30. Chan V, Chan TK, Todd D. Different forms of HbH disease in the Chinese. *Hemoglobin* 1988; 12: 499–507.

31. Embury SH, Miller JA, Dozy AM, Kan YW, Chan V, Todd D: Two different molecular organizations account for the single α-globin gene of the α-thalassemia-2 genotype. *J Clin Invest* 1980; 66: 1319–1325.

32. Ghosh A, Woo JSK, Wan CW, MacHenry C, Wong V, Ma HK, Chan V, Chan TK: Evaluation of a prenatal screening procedure for β-thalassemia carriers in a Chinese population based on the mean corpuscular volume (MCV). *Prenatal Diagnosis* 1985; 5: 59–65.

33. Chan V, Leung NK, Chan TK, Ghosh A, Kan YW, Todd D: BamHI polymorphism in the Chinese: its potential usefulness in prenatal diagnosis of β thalassemia. *Br Med J* 1984; 289: 947–948.

34. Chan V, Chan TK, Cheng MY, Leung NK, Kan YW, Todd D: Characteristics and distribution of β thalassemia haplotypes in South China. *Hum Genet* 1986; 73: 23–26.

35. Chan V, Chan TK, Chehab FF, Todd D: Distribution of β-thalassemia mutations in South China and their association with haplotype. *Am J Hum Genet* 1987; 41: 678–685.

36. Chan V, Chan TK, Ghosh A, Wong LC, Ma HK, Kan YW, Todd D: Application of DNA polymorphisms for prenatal diagnosis of β-thalassemia in Chinese. *Am J Hematol* 1987; 25: 409–415.

37. Chan TK, Chan V, Todd D, Ghosh A, Wong LC, Ma HK: Prenatal diagnosis of α and β thalassemias: experience in Hong Kong. *Hemoglobin* 1988; 12: 787–794.

38. Chan V: Prenatal diagnosis of alpha and beta thalassemia and hemophilia A: experience in Hong Kong. *Clin Biochem* 1989; in press.

39. Chan V, Chan TK, Todd D, Wong LC, Ghosh A, Tang M, Chan FY, Ma HK: Prenatal diagnosis of α and β thalassemias. *Meeting of the Royal College of Pathlogists of Australasia 1989.*

40. Chan V, Chan TK, Todd D, Chan FY, Tang M, Ma HK: Prenatal of thalassemias. *Proc Seminar on First Trimester Prenatal Diagnosis 1988.*

41. Chan V, Chan TK, Kan YW, Todd D: A novel β-thalassemia frameshift mutation (Codon 14/15), detectable by direct visualization of abnormal restriction fragment in amplified genomic DNA. *Blood* 1988; 72: 1420–1423.

42. Chan V, Chan TK, Todd: A new Codon 71 (+T) mutant resulting in β^0 thalassemia. *Blood* 1989 (in press).

43. Chin D, Tse TM, Wong RWS, Todd D, Yu CP, Mann KS: Paraparesis with hemoglobin E-β thalassemia. *Aust NZ J Med* 1985; 15: 263–264.

44. Tso SC: Significance of subnormal red-cell folate in thalassemia. *J Clin Pathol* 1976; 29: 140–143.

45. Tso SC: Folate studies in thalassaemia. *Proc 3rd Meeting Asian Pacific Div, Int Soc Haematol* Jakarta, 1975; 104–105.

46. Tso SC, Chan TK, Todd D: The spleen in haemoglobin H disease. *XVII Cong Int Soc Hematol*, Paris, 1978; 1: 371.

47. Tso SC, Loh TT, Todd D: Iron overload in patients with haemoglobin H disease. *Scand J Haematol* 1984; 32: 391–394.

48. Tso SC, Loh TT, Chen WWC, Wang CCL, Todd D: Iron overload in thalassemic patients in Hong Kong. *Ann Acad Med* 1984; 13: 487–490.

49. Todd D, Chan V. The thalassemias: an update. *Med Progress* 1989 (in press).

50. Todd D: Thalassemia: current concepts in management — Viewpoint from Hong

Kong. *Med Progress* 1976; 3: 17.

51. Lee AKY, Chan V, Chan TK: The identification and localisation of antithrombin III in human tissues. *Thromb Res* 1979; 14: 209–217.

52. Chan V, Chan TK, Wong V, Tso SC, Todd D: The determination of antithrombin III by radioimmunoassay and its clinical application. *Br J Hematol* 1979; 41: 563–572.

53. Chan V, Chan TK: Antithrombin III in fresh and cultural human endothelial cells: a natural anticoagulant from the vascular endothelium. *Thromb Res* 1979; 15: 209–213.

54. Chan TK, Chan V: Antithrombin III, a natural anticoagulant is synthesized by human endothelial cells. *Thromb Haemost* 1981; 46: 504–506.

55. Chan V, Chan TK: Heparin antithrombin III binding: in vitro and in vivo studies. *Haemostasis* 1979; 8: 373–389.

56. Chan TK, Chan V: The effect of venous occlusion on antithrombin III, plasminogen activator and fibrinogen degradation product (Fragment E) levels. *Thromb Res* 1979; 14: 525–534.

57. Tso SC: Deep venous thrombosis after stroke in Chinese. *Aust NZ J Med* 1980; 10: 513–514.

58. Tso SC, Chan TK, Todd D: Venous thrombosis in haemoglobin H disease after splenectomy. *Aust NZ J Med* 1982; 12: 635–638.

59. Tso SC, Wong V, Chan V, Chan TK, Ma HK, Todd D: Deep vein thrombosis and changes in coagulation and fibrinolysis after gynaecological operations in Chinese: the effect of oral contraceptives and malignant diseaase. *Br J Haematol* 1980; 46: 603–612.

60. Wong V, Chan TK, Chan V, Tso SC, Todd D, Ma HK: The effect of oral contraceptives on coagulation and fibrinolytic parameters in the Chinese — A prospective study. *Thromb Haemost* 1982; 48: 263–265.

61. Chan V, Yeung CK, Chan TK: Antithrombin III and fibrinogen degradation product (Fragment E) in diabetic nephropathy. *J Clin Pathol* 1982; 35: 661–666.

62. Chan V, Lai CL, Chan TK: Metabolism of antithrombin III in cirrhosis and carcinoma of the liver. *Clin Sci* 1981; 60: 681–688.

63. Chan TK, Chan GTC; Chan V: Hypofibrinogenaemia due to primary fibrinolysis in two patients with acute promyelocytic leukaemia. *Aust NZ J Med* 1984; 14: 245–249.

64. Chan TK, Chan V, Teng CS, Young RTT: Effets du gliclazide et du glibenclamide sur les fonctions plaquettaires, la fibrinolyse et l'equilibre glycemique chez des diabetiques presentant une retinopathic. *Semaine des Hopitaux de Paris* 1982; 58: 1197–1200.

65. Chan TK, Chan V, Teng CS, Young RTT: Effects du gliclazide et du glibenclamide sur les fonctions plaquettaires, la fibrinolyse et l'equilibre glycemique chez les diabetiques presentant une retinopathie. *J Int de Med* 1984; 9 (Suppl): 67–70.

66. Chan V, Chan TK: Characterization of Factor VIII related protein synthesized by human endothelial cells: a study of structure and function. *Thromb Haemost* 1982; 48: 177–181.

67. Chan V, Chan TK: Cell free synthesis of Factor VIII related protein. *Thromb Haemost* 1983; 50: 835–837.

68. Chan V, Chan TK, Liu VWS, Wong ACK: Restriction fragment length polymorphism associated with Factor VIII: C gene in the Chinese. *Hum Genet* 1988; 79: 128–131.

69. Chan V, Tong TMF, Chan TPT, Tang M, Wan CW, Chan FY, Chu YC, Chan TK: Multiple XbaI polymorphisms for carrier detection and prenatal diagnosis of Haemophilia A. *Br J Haematol* 1989 (in press).

70. Chan TK, Chan V: Prenatal diagnosis of haemophilia. *Proc Seminar on First Trimester Prenatal Diagnosis 1988*.

71. Chan V, Chan TK, Tong TMF, Todd D: A novel missense mutation in exon 4 of the Factor VIII: C gene resulting in moderately severe hemophilia A. *Blood* 1989 (in press).

Vivian CHAN

Research in Haematological Oncology

Introduction

Although haematological malignancies are not the commonest cancer, they have an important impact because of the young average age of the patients. In the past decades, many advances have provided better understanding of the biology of various malignant blood diseases and tremendous success has also been achieved in their treatment. Many of these patients can now enjoy longlasting remissions and apparent cure of the disease. As a leading haematologist, Professor Todd has foreseen and contributed to this development. Together with his other capable colleagues, he has established this Department, many years ago, a major centre for treating and studying various haematological malignancies in Hong Kong. This has provided our unfortunate patients the opportunity of receiving the state-of-art treatment for these diseases. It also facilitates better undergraduate and postgraduate teaching on this subject (1–2). In collaboration with the Department of Pathology and the Institute of Radiotherapy and Oncology, active research has been on-going aiming to study the peculiar pattern of various malignant blood diseases in Hong Kong and to determine the optimal therapy for these patients.

Malignant Lymphomas

About 60–80 new cases of lymphomas are being seen in this Department every year (3). A peculiar pattern of the disease has been recognized (4). Compared to the Caucasian populations, a much lower incidence of Hodgkin's disease and low grade non-Hodgkin's lymphoma is observed in our patients (5–6).

Majority of our patients have intermediate or high grade non-Hodgkin's lymphomas according to the Working Formulation histological classification (4) The Ann Arbor staging classification, B symptoms, age and serum lactate dehydrogenase level have been found to be the most important prognostic factors in these patients (3) Our patients with localized (stage I–II) intermediate grade lymphomas have achieved a 5-year survival of 70% (3). Compared to those receiving radiotherapy alone, these stage I and II patients receiving chemotherapy have fewer relapses. However, their overall survival is similar. This may be due to the effective chemotherapy salvage following radiotherapy failure and the occasional treatment related mortality following chemotherapy (3) For patients with advanced (stage III–IV) intermediate grade lymphomas, 38% of those receiving the CHOP (cyclophosphamide, doxorubicin, vincristine and prednisone) chemotherapy survived beyond 5 years (3, 7–8). The use of the newer regimes, including BACOP and m-BACOD, do not appear to improve further their prognosis (3). High grade non-Hodgkin's lymphomas were characterized by the aggressiveness of the disease and the poorer long term survival (stage I & II: 44%, III & IV: 17%; at 5 years) of these patients. An intensive BACOP/m-BACOD-L17M protocol has been used for our patients with high grade lymphomas and it appears to improve their survival (3). Patients with refractory or relapsing intermediate and high grade lymphomas usually have very poor prognosis, although a small proportion of around 20% may have prolonged remission and survival following salvage chemotherapy (9–10).

Thirty per cent of our cases of intermediate and high grade lymphomas have a T-immunophenotype (3, 11, 12). This figure is higher than the 20% reported in the Caucasian population but lower than the figure of 40–70% observed in Japan. Majority of these cases belong to the group of peripheral T-cell lymphomas but none of them is associated with the human T-cell leukaemia/lymphoma viruses (12). The use of the intensive BACOP/m-BACOD-L17M regime also appears to improve the survival of these patients (12) Compared to their B-cell counterparts, peripheral T-cell lymphoma is associated with an increased incidence of systemic B symptoms but a lower incidence of bulky disease (3). Also, the disease tends to affect more commonly liver, spleen, bone marrow, nasal region and skin (3). However, the immunophenotype does not appear to affect the prognosis (3).

Our lymphoma patients appear to have a

high incidence of extranodal disease (3, 4). The gastrointestinal tract, the nasal region and the Waldeyer's ring are the common primary sites outside the lymph nodes (13–18). These lymphomas all have their own distinctive features (3).

The peculiar pattern of lymphomas in Hong Kong Chinese is interesting. This is being studied further in this Department and the Department of Pathology using the modern techniques in molecular biology aiming to obtain a better understanding of the biology of lymphomas (19).

Leukaemia

Majority of our leukaemia patients are suffering from acute myeloid leukaemia (AML) (20–23). The use of an induction regime consisting of cytarabine and doxorubicin has resulted in long-term remission in 20–25% of our AML patients (24). In association with the Australian Leukaemia Study Group, a more intensive regime consisting of cytarabine, doxorubicin and etoposide has been investigated (25). Compared to a similar regime but without etoposide, this intensive regime is more toxic but has resulted in longer disease-free survival in the subgroup of younger patients. For our patients with refractory or recurrent AML, the prognosis is poor. Only 24% of these patients respond to our salvage treatment consisting of cytarabine, thioguanine and amsacrine and those with a previous remission longer than six months have a significantly better chance of responding. However, most of these responses are only of short duration (26).

Unlike children, only a small proportion of our leukaemic patients have acute lymphoblastic leukaemia (ALL) and our treatment results for adult ALL are disappointing. Our UMU-ALL-I protocol used between 1978 to 1984 has resulted in a median survival of only 12 months and late relapses are seen many years following remissions (27). A more intensive UMU-ALL-II protocol has been used between 1984 and 1987. It results in a median survival of 13 months only and does not appear to improve the prognosis of our ALL patients (28). The causes of these poor treatment results are reviewed. Compared to literature, it appears that a higher proportion of our ALL patients belong to the poor prognostic groups of male sex, elderly age, null-cell immunophenotype and high initial white cell count.

However, this cannot totally account for our poor treatment results, as our ALL patients in the so-called good-prognosis subgroups apparently do not do well either (28).

Other malignant blood diseases including chronic myeloid leukaemia, myelodysplastic syndrome and myeloma are also being studied and treated in this Department (29–31).

Toxicities of Chemotherapy

Reversible depression of bone marrow is an inevitable event of cytotoxic chemotherapy. In the management of haematological malignancies, deliberate attempts are made to produce periods of neutropenia in order to maximize the efficacy of therapy, resulting in an increased risk of opportunistic infection. Prophylactic oral antibiotic such as co-trimoxazole has been recommended to prevent bacterial as well as pneumocystis infections in neutropenic patients. However, bacterial resistance and drug toxicities associated with co-trimoxazole are troublesome. Ofloxacin, an oral fluorinated quinolone, has been shown in our randomized study to be more superior than co-trimoxazole in preventing gram-negative infection in neutropenic patients following chemotherapy and is associated with fewer toxicities (32) However, co-trimoxazole is probably still useful as a pneumocystis prophylaxis. For those who develop bacterial infection during the neutropenic period, intravenous combination antibiotics are effective in reducing morbidity and mortality. However, these combinations which often contain aminoglycoside are potentially toxic. We have shown in a pilot study that imipenem, a new antibiotic, with a wide spectrum of antibacterial activity, when used alone is a practical alternative to antibiotic combinations in treating neutropenic infection (33) Prospective randomized study is on-going to compare this drug with ceftazidime which has also been shown to be effective as a monotherapy for neutropenic infection.

Compared to the 10% hepatitis B surface antigen (HBsAg) carrier rate in the general population, a higher figure of 22% of our lymphoma patients are found to be HBsAg positive at the time of initial diagnosis (3). This may be related to the immunosuppressive effect of lymphoma. Up to 21% of our HbsAg positive lymphoma patients develop reactivation of the hepatitis B infection during therapy for their lymphoma and some are fatal (3, 37). There is no reliable factor predicting its development and ways of prevention are being investigated (3).

Late chemotherapeutic toxicity has become an important problem as more and more patients with various haematological malignancies are cured of their diseases. The effect of combination chemotherapy on the pituitary-gonadal function has been studied in our patients with leukaemia and lymphoma (35). Sterility is related to chemotherapy especially those regimes containing alkylating agents. The gonadal damage is also not restricted to the germinal tissue (35, 36).

Patients with malignant blood diseases are facing a difficult battle. The unpleasant side effects and the long duration of therapy often result in considerable psychological stress. Social and financial problems are not uncommonly encountered. Sympathetic support from the management team is of utmost importance (37).

Epilogue

The prognosis of patients with malignant blood diseases has markedly improved with the advances in therapy. However, the optimal treatment for various categories of patients remains to be defined. Less toxic treatment is needed by patients with responsive diseases and more effective therapy has to be developed for those with refractory or relapsed illnesses. Many innovative treatments have been developed recently. Bone marrow transplantation has been shown to play an important role in the management of malignant blood diseases. With the opening of the new Queen Mary Hospital extension, we hope we will be able to perform our first marrow transplantation soon.

References

1. Ng RP, Todd D: Management of malignant lymphoma: a brief review. *Bull HKMA* 1977; 29: 13–20.
2. Liang R, Todd D: Current Management of non-Hodgkin's lymphoma. *Medical Progress* 1987; 14: 17–28.
3. Liang R: Malignant lymphomas in Hong Kong Chinese. M. D. thesis, University of Hong Kong, 1989.
4. Ho FCS, Todd D, Loke SL, Ng RP, Khoo R: Clinicopathological features of malignant lymphomas in 294 Hong Kong Chinese patients — Retrospective study covering an eight year period. *Int J Cancer* 1984; 34: 143–148.
5. Liang R, Choi P, Todd D, Chan TK, Choy D, Ho F: Hodgkin's disease in Hong Kong Chinese. *Hematol Oncol* (in press).
6. Liang R, Todd D, Chan TK, Ng RP, Choy D, Loke SL, Ho FCS: Follicular non-Hodgkin's lymphoma in Hong Kong Chinese: a retrospective analysis. *Hematol Oncol* 1988; 6: 29–37.
7. Ng RP, Todd D, Ho FCS, Khoo RKK: Histiocytic diffuse non-Hodgkin's lymphoma (abstr). *International Society of Haematology, Asian Pacific Division, 4th Meeting, Seoul, Korea*, 1979; p. 42.
8. Ng RP, Todd D, Khoo RKK, Ho FCS: Combination chemotherapy in non-Hodgkin's lymphoma. *Annual Meeting, Haematology Society of Australia and Australasian Society of Blood Transfusion, Hobart, 1979.*
9. Ng RP, Todd D, Khoo RKK: Salvage chemotherapy for non-Hodgkin's lymphoma. *Cancer Treat Rep* 1982; 66: 1977–1979.
10. Liang R, Todd D, Chan TK: HOAP-Bleo as salvage therapy for diffuse aggressive non-Hodgkin's lymphoma. *Cancer Chemother Pharmacol* 1988; 22: 169–172.
11. Ho FCS, Loke SL, Hui PK, Todd D: Immunohistological subtypes of non-Hodgkin's lymphomas in Hong Kong Chinese. *Pathology* 1986; 18: 426–430.
12. Liang R, Todd D, Chan TK, Wong KL, Ho F, Loke SL: Peripheral T cell lymphoma. *J Clin Oncol* 1987; 5: 759–765.
13. Liang R, Kay R, Maisey MN: Brachial plexus infiltration by non-Hodgkin's lymphoma. *Br J Radiol* 1985; 58: 1125–1127.
14. Liang R, Todd D, Chan TK, Ng RP, Ho FCS: Gastrointestinal lymphoma in Chinese: a retrospective analysis. *Hematol Oncol* 1987; 5: 115–126.
15. Liang R, Ng RP, Todd D, Choy D, Khoo RKK, Ho FCS: Management of stage I–II

diffuse aggressive non-Hodgkin's lymphoma of the Waldeyer's ring: combined modality therapy versus radiotherapy alone. *Hematol Oncol* 1987; 5: 223–230.

16. Chung HT, Wong KL, Liang RHS, Loke SL, Liu HW, Tso WK, Chan SCH, Lam KSL, Lai CL: Non-Hodgkin's lymphoma as a cause of hypoadrenalism. *Aust N Z J Med* 1987; 17: 605–607.

17. Liang R, Woo E, Ho F, Collins R, Choy D, Ma J: Klinefelter's syndrome and primary central nervous system lymphoma. *Med Ped Oncol* (in press).

18. Liang R, Woo E, Yu YL, Todd D, Chan TK, Ho FCS, Tso SC, Shum JST: Central nervous system involvement by non-Hodgkin's lymphoma. *Eur J Cancer Clin Oncol* 1989; 25: 703–710.

19. Liang R, Chan V, Chan TK, Todd D, Ho F, Choi P: Gene rearrangement of peripheral blood and bone marrow: lymphoma of mucosa-associated lymphoid tissue. *The 25th Annual Meeting of the American Society of Clinical Oncology, USA, May, 1989*, No. 1014.

20. Woo E, Yue CP, Mann KS, Cheung FMF, Chan TK, Todd D: Intracerebral choromas. *Clin Neurol Neurosurg* 1986; 88: 135–139.

21. Ho FSC, Chan GTC, Todd D: Nonspecificity of Sudan Black in the diagnosis of acute myeloid leukaemia. *Br J Haematol* 1983; 53: 171–172.

22. Chan TK, Chan GTC, Chan V: Hypofibriongenaemia due to increased fibrinolysis in two patients with acute promyelocytic leukaemia. *Aust NZJ Med* 1984; 14: 245–249.

23. Liu HW, Wong KL, Chan TYK, Lau CC, Liang R: Superior vena cava syndrome: a rare presenting feature of acute myeloid leukaemia. *Acta Haematol* 1988; 79: 213–216.

24. Tso SC, Lee AKY, Chan TK, Ng RP, Todd D: Extended induction therapy in adult myeloid leukaemia with cytarabine and doxorubicin and the effect of levamisole (abstr). *International Society of Haematology, Asian-Pacific Division, 4th Meeting, Seoul, Korea, 1979*; p. 70.

25. Australian Leukaemia Study Group. Etoposide for remission induction of adult acute nonlymphocytic leukaemia (abstr). *4th International Symposium on Therapy of Acute Leukaemia, Rome, Italy, 1987*; p. 112.

Bishop JF, Lowenthal RM, Joshua D, Matthews JP, Todd D, Cobcroft R, Whiteside MG, Kronenberg H, Ma D, Dodds A, Herrmann R, Szer J, Wolf MM, Young G, for the Australian Leukemia Study Group (ALSG): Etoposide in acute non-lymphocytic leukemia. *Blood* 1989 (in press).

26. Liang R, Chan TK, Todd D: Chemotherapy for relapsed and resistant acute nonlymphoblastic leukaemia. *Cancer Chemother Pharmacol* 1988; 21: 68–70.

27. Cheng PNM, Tso SC, Chan TK, Todd D, Lawton JWM, Ho FCS: Acute lymphoblastic leukaemia in Chinese adults in Hong Kong. *Aust NZ J Med* 1989; 19: 37–43.

28. Liang R, Chan TK, Chan GTC, Todd D: Treatment of adult acute lymphoblastic leukaemia using an intensive chemotherapy protocol. *Cancer Chemother Pharmacol* 1989; 23: 384–388.

29. Chiu EKW, Ganeshaguru K, Hoffbrand AV, Mehta AB: Circulating monoclonal B lymphocytes in multiple myeloma. *Br J Haematol* 1989; 72: 28–31

30. Woo E, Yu YL, Ng M, Huang CY, Todd D: Spinal cord compression in multiple myeloma, who gets it? *Aust NZ J Med* 1986; 16: 671–675.

31. Lin CK, Liang R, Fu KH, Ma L, Tse PWT, Chan GTC, Liu HW: Myelodysplastic syndrome presenting with generalised cutaneous granulocytic sarcoma. *Acta Haematol* (in press).

32. Liang R, Yung RWH, Chan TK, Chau PY, Lam WK, So SY, Todd D: Ofloxacin versus co-trimoxazole for prevention of infection in neutropenic patients. *Antimicrob Agents Chemother* (in press).

33. Liang R, Yung R, Chan PY, Chan TK, Lam WK, So SY, Todd D: Imipenem/Cilastatin as initial therapy for febrile neutropenic patients. *J Antimicrob Chemother* 1988; 22: 765–770.

34. Lau JYN, Lai CL, Lin HJ, Lok ASF, Liang RHS, Wu PC, Chan TK, Todd D: Fatal reactivation of chronic hepatitis B virus infection following chemotherapy withdrawal in lymphoma patients. *Q J Med* (in press).

35. Wang CCL, Ng RP, Chan TK, Todd D: Effect of combination chemotherapy on pituitary-gonadal function in patients with lymphoma and leukaemia. *Cancer* 1980; 45:

2030–2037.

36. Wang CCL, Ng RP, Chan TK, Todd D: Leydig cell dysfunction after combination chemotherapy. *Lancet* 1981; ii: 529.

37. Shuen SP, Liang R: Treatment of cancer: a patient's description. *J HKMA* 1988; 40: 70–72.

Raymond H.S. LIANG

ACHIEVEMENTS IN IMMUNOLOGY/RHEUMATOLOGY

Immunology and Rheumatology is a relatively new discipline within the Department of Medicine. This was initially founded by Drs. A.K.Y. Lee and L.W. Mak and later joined by Drs. R.W.S. Wong (Rheumatology), K.L. Wong (Immunology/Rheumatology) and K.H. Chan (Rheumatology).

Research

Between 1975–1978, Dr. Mak had set up techniques in complement component analysis and the application of this technology to study the complement profile in various clinical situation. Dr. A. Lee established the facilities for lymphocyte cultures for studies of cell-mediated immunity. Further studies in the immunological aspect of HBsAg in different clinical conditions was continued.

Unfortunately, both Drs. Lee and Mak left the Department in 1979. Despite their regular attendance at outpatient clinics and Dr. Lee at the weekly Rheumatology Rounds, the development of Clinical Immunology/Rheumatology as a research discipline came to a halt.

Dr. C. K. Yeung, the nephrologist of our Department, had also contributed significantly to the management and research in lupus glomerulonephritis with main emphasis on the survival, response to treatment, tubular dysfunction and $\beta 2$ microglobular level in this condition.

Prospective studies on various clinical aspects in SLE was initiated from Feb 1985 which included the pattern of SLE in Hong Kong Chinese, neurological manifestation of lupus, lupus pregnancies, opportunistic infection etc. Most of the study were completed by Feb 1989 and now in the process of preparation for submission to international journals. In the laboratory, immunogenetic studies in SLE was finished by 1986, studies on soluble interleukin-2 receptor was completed by Sept 1989 and on going research project included T cell receptor gene and immunoglobulin gene rearrangement and anticardiolipin antibodies in SLE.

Immunoregulation in patients with hepatitis B related disease was also established using an in vitro method since February 1985. In line with the same model, immunological changes associated with adoptive immunotherapy with interleukin-2 and lymphokine-activated killer cells in hepatocellular carcinoma was also studied.

A formal aphersis unit was established with Prof. T.K. Chan in March 1985 and the Clinical Immunology Service was in charge of the unit. The unit was responsible to organize and perform all the apheresis procedure. Various disease over these years was treated by plasma exchange and a number of studies was initiated which included its efficacy in treatment of neurological disorders, hypercholesterolemia, SLE, retinal vasculitis etc. A prospective study on the complication, especially infection, was also established at about the same time.

Collaboration was made with Department of Clinical Immunology, Department of Pathology and Department of Obstetrics & Gynaecology on the study of the immunological aspect of various diseases or clinical situation: initially Dr. Mak with Dr. J. Lawton in the immunological changes in pregnancy and trophoblastic diseases, Dr. Lee in the vertical transmission of hepatitis B infections. After Feb 1985, studies were preformed with Dr. B. Jones for the patients with common variable immunodeficiency, or other primary immunodeficiency syndrome, isolated IgA deficiency in patients with SLE, circulating interleukin-2 inhibitor in patients with refractory tuberculosis. Studies on anti-neutrophil cytoplasmic antibodies in Wegener's granulomatosis and SLE was performed with Dr. J.W.M. Lawton.

Research into other rheumatic diseases are scanty and would need much more efforts.

Clinical Service

The subspecialty is responsible to take care of patients with immunodeficiency syndromes, SLE, rheumatoid arthritis, vasculitis and various rheumatic diseases.

A clinical service clinic for Immunology/Rheumatology was established years before Lupus Nephritis Clinic was set up in 1983, primary

Immunodeficiency Clinic and Vasculitis Clinic in 1986.

A joint consultation clinic with Department of Orthopaedics was established and improves the communication between the Rheumatologist and the Surgeon.

The subspecialty was also in charge of performing all apheresis procedures and regular plasma exchange were carried out since March 1985.

Teaching

Undergraduates. This consisted of initially 4 systemic lectures in the beginning of 1974–1975 and now 6 systemic lectures. There were about 3–4 teaching clinics per year.
Elective students were taken for their rotation in this specialty at roughly one per year.

Postgraduate. We are responsible to take trainee in our Department on a regular rotation basis. We also accept medical officers from other hospital for clinical attachment to our subspecialty — approximately one per year.

Development and publications. Because of the limitation of time and manpower, a lot of clinical material and data were available but pending preparation for publication. Though the Department has offered much, the development of this discipline is slow. More opportunities should be given to the trainee and allow them to have training work on the clinical and the laboratory aspects. Study of allergy as a discipline should be established.

Publications in Preparation

1. Wong KL, Hawkins BR, Wong RWS, Dunckley H, Serjeantson SW, Cheng IKP, Chan KH: Immunogenetics in Chinese patients with systemic lupus erythematosus.
2. Wong KL: Danazol in treatment of lupus thrombocytopenia.
3. Wong KL: Dapsone in treatment of cutaneous vasculitis in patient with systemic lupus erythematosus.
4. Wong KL, Yung RWH, Wong WS, So SY: Nocardiosis in patients with systemic lupus erythematosus.
5. Wong KL, Liu HW, Ho KMT, Wong WS: Prevalence and clinical significance of lupus anticoagulant and anticardiolipin antibody in Chinese patients with SLE.
6. Wong KL, Chan SWF, Wong R: Plasmapheresis in patients with acute severe SLE.
7. Wong KL, Cheng IKP, Chan KW, Wong WS, Chan PCK: Membranous lupus nephropathy.
8. Wong KL, Yeung CK, Cheng IKP, Chan KW, Chan MK, Wong WS, Chan PCK: Crescentic lupus glomerulonephritis — Revisited.
9. Wong KL, Ip M, Ngan H, Lam WK, Chan F: Abnormal chest radiograph in patients with SLE.
10. Wong KL, Wong WS, Cheng IKP, Ng MT, Lau YN, Chung HT, Lai CL: Protein losing enteropathy in patients with SLE or related disease.
11. Wong KL, So SY, Ip M, Lam WK, Yuen KY: Mycobaterial infection in SLE.
12. Wong KL: Fatal opportunistic infection in SLE.
13. Wong KL, Jones BM: The immunological dysfunction of isolated IgA deficiency in patients with SLE.
14. Chen RYL, Wong KL, Jones BM, Lawton JWM, Ho FCS: Using streptavidin-biotin-peroxidase complex for the detection of antinuclear antibodies on HEp 2-substrate.
15. Chen RYL, Wong KL, Jones BM, Lawton JWM, Ho FCS: HEp-2 cell substrate for antinuclear screening: Hong Kong experience.
16. Chen RYL, Wong KL, Jones BM, Lawton JWM, Ho FCS: Clinical appraisal of antinuclear antibodies detection using streptavidin-biotin-peroxidase complex on HEp 2 cells.
17. Wong KL: Limitation of serum soluble interleukin-2 receptor in defining the activity of SLE.
18. Wong KL, Chan FY, Lee CP: Outcome of pregnancy in patients with SLE: a prospective study.
19. Wong KL, Woo EKW, Yu YL, Wong RWS: Neurological manifestation of SLE: a prospective study.
20. Leung WH, Wong KL, Lau CP, Wong CK: Cheung CH, Tai YT: Doppler Echocardi-

ographic evaluation of left ventricular diastolic function in patients with SLE.

21. Wong KL: Pulse methyl prednisolone therapy in the treatment of acute refractory lupus thrombocytopenia.

22. Wong KL, Lam CM: Vaso-occlusive retinal vasculitis in SLE.

23. Wong KL, Jones BM, Lawton JWM: Pattern of SLE in Hong Kong Chinese: a retrospective and prospective study.

24. Wong KL, Lam CM, Wong RWS: Ophthalmic complications in patients with SLE: a retrospetive and prospective study.

25. Wong KL, Woo EKW, So SY, Lam WK, Ip M, Yu YL: Plasmapheresis in treatment of ventilator dependent anticholinergic receptor antibody negative myasthenia gravis.

26. Wong KL, Woo EKW, So SY, Lam WK, Ip M, Yu YL, Choy D: Total lymphoid irradiation in treatment of plasmapheresis dependent myasthenia gravis.

27. Wong KL, Jones BM: Common variable immunodeficiency in Hong Kong Chinese.

28. Wong KL, Jones BM, So SY, Lam WK: Circulating interleukin-2 inhibitor and soluble interleukin-2 receptor in refactory tuberculosis.

29. Wong KL, Lee KLF, Chan BCH: Desentization of rifampicin induced toxic hepatiits.

30. Wong KL, Tsui EYL, Ip M, Yuen KY: Erythromycin in the treatment of refractory tuberculosis.

31. Wong KL, Jones BM, Ip M, Kwan SYL: Plasmapheresis in the treatment of refractory tuberculosis and circulating interleukin-2 inhibitor.

32. Wong KL, Lawton JWM, So SY, Ip M: Wegener's granulomatosus in Hong Kong Chinese.

33. Wong KL, Woo EKW, Yu YL, Huang CY: Vasculitic neuropathy.

Publications

1. Lee AKY: Hepatitis B antigen and autoantibodies in chronic liver disease in Hong Kong. *Aust NZ J Med* 1975 Jun; 5: 235–239.

2. Chan WC, Ng WL, Lee AKY, Yu RYH: Lupus nephritis in Hong Kong. *Ann Acad Med Singapore* 1975 Apr; 4(2): 58–65.

3. Lee AKY, Eisinger M: Cell-mediated immunity (CMI) to human wart virus and wart-associated tissue antigens. *Clin Exp Immunol* 1976; 26: 419–424.

4. Mak LW, Lachmann PJ, Majewski J: Techniques of fractionating complement in vivo by the use of activated complement components to trigger to C3b feedback cycle. *J Immunol* 1976; 116: 1741.

5. Mak LW: Complement technology in clinical medicines. *Journal of the Hong Kong Medical Technology Association* 1977; 2(3): 11–23.

6. Mak LW, Lachmann PJ, Majewski J: The activation of the C3b feedback cycle with human complement components. I. Through the classical pathway. *Clin Exp Immunol* 1977; 30: 200–210.

7. Mak LW, Majewsky J, Lachmann PJ: The activation of the C3b feedback cycle with human complement components. II. Using components of the alternative pathway. *Clin Exp Immunol* 1977; 30: 211–221.

8. Lawton JWM, Lo NS, Sin WK, Buchanan AJC, Mak LW: Idiopathic late-onset immunoglobulin deficiency with associated defect in cell-mediated immunity. *Arch Dis Child* 1977; 52: 899–901.

9. Lam KC, Lai CL, Lee AKY: Presenting clinical features of HBsAg-positive liver cirrhosis in Chinese. *Gastroenterology* 1977; 73: A–21.

10. Lee AKY, Chan Vivian NY, Chan TK: The identification and localization of antithrombin III in human tissues. *Thromb Res* 1979; 14: 209–217.

11. Mak LW. The complement profile in relation to the 'reactor' state: a study in the immediate post-partum period. *Immunology* 1978 Mar; 31: 419–425.

12. Ho PC, Mak LW, Lawton JWM, Ma HK: Immunological parameters in gestational trophoblastic neoplasia. *J Reprod Immunol* 1980; 1: 307–319.

13. Wong Vivian CW; Lee AKY, Ip Henrietta MH: Transmission of hepatitis B antigens from symptom free carrier mothers to the fetus and the infant. *Br J Obstet Gynaecol* 1980 Nov; 87: 958–965.

14. Ho PC, Mak LW, Lawton JWM: Immunology parameters in pregnancy. *Afr J Clin Immunol* 1981; 2: 25–32.

15. Lee AKY: Systemic lupus erythematosus in

Hong Kong. *Hong Kong Practitioner* 1982; 4(2): 49–53.

16. Lee AKY: Rheumatoid arthritis: problems in management. *Medical Progress* 1983; 10(6): 17–24.

17. Mak LW: Drug treatment of rheumatoid arthritis. *Hong Kong Practitioner* 1982 Mar; 4(3): 77–81.

18. Yeung CK, Wong KL, Ng RP, Ng WL: Tubular dysfunction in SLE. *Nephron* 1984; 36: 84–88.

19. Yeung CK, Wong KL, Wong WS, Ng MT, Chan KW, Ng WL: Crescentic lupus glomerulonephritis. *Clin Nephrol* 1984; 21(5): 251–258.

20. Yeung CK, Wong KL, Wong RWS, Chan MK, Ng WL: Unusual transformations of renal involvement in systemic lupus erythematosus. *Aust NZ J Med* 1985; 15: 69–71.

21. Wong KL, Gibson J, Basten A: Maternal autoimmune disease influences self-tolerance in offspring. In *Micro-environments in the Lymphoid System* (ed. Klaus GGB), Plenum Publishing Corporation, 1985; pp. 495–502.

22. Wong KL, Basten A, Gibson J, Loblay RH, Fazeka de St Groth B: The role of memory suppressor T cells in self-tolerance: induction in utero and in athymic mice. In *Micro-environments in the Lymphoid System* (ed. Klaus GGB), Plenum Publishing Corporation, 1985; pp. 511–520.

23. Yeung CK, Ng WL, Wong RWS, Wong KL, Chan MK: Acute deterioration in renal function in systemic lupus erythematosus. *Q J Med* 1985 Jul; 56(219): 393–402.

24. Yeung CK, Wong KL, Wong WS, Chan KH: β2-microglobulin and systemic lupus erythematosus. *J Rheumatol* 1986; 13(6): 1053–1058.

25. Wong KL, Tai YT, Loke SL, Woo EKW, Wong WS, Chan MK, Ma J: Disseminated zygomycosis masquerading as cerebral lupus erythematosus. *Am J Pathol* 1986; 86(4): 546–549.

26. Kumana CR, Chan Maureen MY, Wong KL, Wong RWS, Kou M: Frequency distribution of acetylator phenotypes in Hong Kong systemic lupus erythematosus patients and controls (Abstract). *The Tenth International Congress of Pharmacology in Sydney, Australia*, No. 0239 (August 1987).

27. Yu YL, Woo EKW, Wong KL, Tse BSS, Lau YN: Cryptococcal infection of the nervous system. *Q J Med* 1988; 66: 87–96.

28. Wong RWS, Chan JKH, Wong KL: Lupus anticoagulant — A double misnomer. *Asian Pacific Journal of Allergy and Immunology* 1987; 5: 161–165.

29. Kwong YL, Wong KL, Kung ITM, Chan PCK, Lam WK: Concomitant alveolar haemorrhage and cytomegalovirus infection in a patient with systemic lupus erythematosus. *Postgrad Med J* 1988; 64: 56–59.

30. Hawkins BR, Wong KL, Wong RWS, Chan KH, Dunckley H, Seyeantson SW: Strong association between the major histocompatibility complex and SLE in Southern Chinese. *J Rheumatol* 1987; 14(6): 1128–1131.

31. Liu HW, Wong KL, Lin CK, Wong WS, Tse PWT, Chan GTC: The reapprasial of dilute tissue thromboplastin inhibition test in the diagnosis of lupus anticoagulant. *Br J Haematol* 1989; 72: 229–234.

32. Leung WH, Wong KL, Lau CP, Wong CK, Cheung CH, So KF: Myocardial involvement in Chung-Strauss Syndrome — the role of endomyocardial biopsy. *J Rheumatol* 1989; 16: 828–831.

K.L. WONG

ACHIEVEMENTS IN NEUROLOGY

Neurology is a relatively young subspecialty in the Department of Medicine. Prior to 1981, Dr. M. Lee, an honorary member of the staff, undertook the responsibility of neurology teaching and clinical service on a limited scale. Since its inception in 1981, the Neurology Service has been staffed by Dr. C.Y. Huang (1981 to 1986), Dr. Y.L. Yu (1983 to date), Dr. D. Chin (1984), Dr. E. Woo (1985 to 1988), Dr. Y.W. Chan (1985) and Dr. C.M. Chang (1989 to date). The main activities are clinical service, teaching and research of neurological diseases.

Clinical Service

The Neurology Service is based at Queen Mary Hospital and Tung Wah Hospital. All the acute cases are admitted into Queen Mary Hospital where there is a full range of facilities including Neuroradiology, Neurosurgery and Clinical Neurophysiology. About 4000 patients are admitted annually, 40% with stroke, 15% with epilepsy and the rest exhibiting the full spectrum of neurological disorders. The subacute and chronic cases are admitted into Tung Wah Hospital, which has a comprehensive Stroke Rehabilitation Unit and a Laboratory for Clinical Neurophysiology. About 500 patients are admitted annually, the majority being stroke victims. In addition, approximately 10 new and 130 old cases are seen at the Sai Ying Pun Jockey Club Clinic each week. Over the years, the Service has established a solid reputation in patient care and has become the major referral centre for patients with neurological diseases. Plans for expansion are underway. A purpose-designed Neurology Ward at Queen Mary Hospital will be opened in 1992 and the Neurodiagnostic Laboratory at Tung Wah Hospital will be enlarged to accommodate new facilities for assessment and treatment of extrapyramidal disorders.

Education

Vigorous teaching programmes for undergraduates and postgraduates are operative. The modes of teaching for medical students are lectures, clinics and bedside sessions. Postgraduate training is given in ward rounds, 3-monthly neurological rotations and weekly Neurology meetings. Joint scientific meetings with the Hong Kong Neurology Society are also held regularly. These meetings are well-attended by neurologists, neurosurgeons, radiologists and trainees in Neurology and Internal Medicine. In recent years, there has been a substantial improvement in the standard of Neurology among students and a much greater awareness among practitioners of the service which is offered by neurologists.

In addition, teaching is also undertaken for dental students, postgraduates of the Clinical Psychology course, and in the near future, students of the Speech and Hearing Sciences course. Education of patients and the lay public is carried out via information leaflets on major neurological diseases like stroke and epilepsy. Staff members of this Department took an advisory role in the recent public health exhibition entitled 'The Nervous System — A Perspective' organized by our students.

Research

The emphasis of neurological research has been clinical, since the disease patterns and normal values among the local population had not previously been documented. The data acquired so far have provided insight into clinical management and have laid the groundwork for further research on neurological disorders in the local population. Because of the shortages of resources and suitably trained staff, research in more basic aspects of neurological disorders has been undertaken on a relatively small scale in collaboration with scientist colleagues. For example, genetic factors in multiple sclerosis and myasthenia gravis are being investigated (with Dr. B.R. Hawkins, Department of Pathology).

Major Research Projects

1.   Cerebrovascular disease. Stroke is the most

common neurological disease, the third leading cause of mortality and the main source of disability in the elderly. Thus, our main efforts have been directed to this area. A Stroke Data Bank has been established, with accurate documentation of stroke subtypes, risk factors and outcome. An important finding is that lacunar infarct and deep cerebral haemorrhage, which reflect small cerebral vessel disease, are more prevalent in Hong Kong Chinese compared with the Caucasoid populations. We have also clarified the issue that a high glucose level at admission, rather than a cause for poor outcome, is in fact a stress response to a bad stroke. The clinical picture and the underlying pathology of the various lacunar syndromes, 'cerebral steal' from arteriovenous malformations, and subcortical arteriosclerotic encephalopathy have been delineated. The beta-thromboglobulin level has been shown to be elevated in thrombo-embolic infarcts rather than lacunar infarcts, thus reaffirming the important role of platelet aggregation in the former condition. These efforts have supplied much needed data as well as direction to subsequent stroke research. As a result, rigorous clinical trials on treatments of acute stroke are now taking place.

2. Dysphasia in the Chinese. Chinese is an ideogram language, as opposed to English which is a phonemic language. The language disorders in the Chinese are therefore substantially different from those in English-speaking subjects. Stroke affecting the speech area in the dominant cerebral hemisphere is not uncommon and thus provides ample opportunities for the systematic study of dysphasia. The pioneer work of an Assessment Battery for Chinese Dysphasics has been completed and a number of theoretical issues have been identified.

3. Spinal cord disorders. Apart from trauma, cervical spondylotic myelopathy is the most common cervical spinal cord lesion in the middle-aged or above. The clinical picture, pathogenetic mechanisms and the roles of somatosensory evoked potentials and computed tomography in this condition have been elucidated. A related condition, known

as ossification of the posterior longitudinal ligament, has also been thoroughly investigated. In both conditions, the sagittal diameter of the cervical spinal canal is the crucial factor for cord damage and control values for the Chinese population have been established. A project to determine the recovery of neural function following surgical treatment is in progress with the collaboration of the Departments of Physiology and Orthopaedic Surgery.

4. Multiple sclerosis (MS). A territory-wide investigation of this disease has been completed. It is a rare disease in Hong Kong Chinese, with a prevalence of 0. 88 per million population. This figure is similar to other Oriental populations but much lower than in Caucasoids. The symptomatology and the clinical course are however the same as elsewhere. Compared with Caucasoid patients, two further differences exist, viz. a low detection rate of oligoclonal immunoglobulin in the cerebrospinal fluid, and a lack of association with Human Leucocyte Antigens (HLA), DR2 or others, at the serological level. Based on these observations, a hypothesis on the still uncertain pathogenesis of MS has been proposed. We postulate that genetic factors coded within the Major Histocompatibility Complex determine the response of the central nervous system to immunological challenge. We believe the genes are related to those determining a variant of HLA-DR2. The Chinese are less genetically susceptible to MS and hence develop abnormal immune responses to a much smaller extent. To test this hypothesis, DNA analysis of the HLA-DR2 antigen is in progress and the preliminary results are encouraging.

5. Myasthenia gravis (MG). The Myasthenia Gravis Research Group was formed in 1986 to launch a territory-wide study. This work has generated a comprehensive Data Bank on MG. The similarities of the disease in Hong Kong Chinese with Caucasoid patients include a prevalence of 63 per million and an incidence of 4 per million population, a low familial occurrence, female predominance in adult patients and the clinical features. The distinct features of MG in Hong

Kong Chinese are the lack of female predominance in paediatric patients, a single peak for the age of onset in the first three decades, the higher proportion of paediatric patients and restricted ocular disease. Moreover, the detection rate of acetylcholine receptor antibody in our patients is low, and there is a strong association with the HLA-DR9 antigen. These two observations are particularly obvious in juvenile onset MG with restricted ocular involvement. Such data support the argument for different clinical expressions of MG in different racial groups, and there is good evidence that these are genetically determined. Further analysis of the HLA-DR9 antigen at the DNA level is currently in progress.

6. Epilepsy. This is a common neurological problem affecting mainly young people in their formative and productive years. Effective control of seizures with anticonvulsants is now possible. Our research has specifically addressed the issue of therapeutic drug levels and seizure control. Consequently, we recommend that drug level is secondary in importance to clinical observations of seizure frequency and the presence of side effects. The long-term effects of phenytoin on neural function have also been studied by recording brain stem auditory evoked potentials. It is concluded that phenytoin exerts a subclinical peripheral effect (at the cochlear and auditory nerve) as well as a central effect (at the brain stem), particularly when administered at high dosages.

7. Infections. Infection of the central nervous system remains a serious and relatively common problem, even though effective modern antimicrobials are available. Opportunistic infections have become more prevalent because of the increasing number of immunocompromised patients, either due to the disease *per se* or drug therapy. Yet the diagnosis of these infections can be elusive. For these reasons, we have documented the clinical picture of two opportunistic infections, namely cryptococcosis and tuberculosis. Furthermore, we have discovered that a relatively common bacterial meningitis in Hong Kong is occupation-related. *Streptococcus suis*

meningitis is more liable to occur in subjects whose occupations are associated with handling pigs or pork. It has the same clinical features as other acute bacterial meningitides but severe bilateral deafness is an almost invariable complication.

8. Neoplasms. The nervous system is frequently the secondary site of involvement by other malignancies. We have studied the characteristics of spinal cord and root involvement in patients with multiple myeloma. In the Chinese, non-Hodgkin's lymphoma is more common than Hodgkin's lymphoma and we have documented the varieties and outcome of neurological involvement. Nasopharyngeal carcinoma is a common malignancy locally and at an early stage, it is largely curable with radiotherapy. However, the long-term effect of radiotherapy on the brain, and especially on the temporal lobes and hypothalamic-pituitary axis, is a serious yet hitherto little described complication. We have brought this to the attention of practitioners and recommended means to reduce the incidence and severity of this complication.

Future Plans

Apart from a contribution to world literature, the above projects and other smaller ones have generated a solid data base on neurological diseases in Hong Kong. The differences in disease patterns and characteristics between our population and others, in particular the Caucasoids, have provided us with greater insight into the pathogenesis and causations of these diseases. We are now poised to embark on larger scale clinical research into problems relevant to Hong Kong, and to collaborate with basic scientists in laboratory research. With regard to the latter, the major areas identified are 'Genetic factors in neurological diseases' (with Dr. V. Chan, Department of Medicine and Dr. B.R. Hawkins, Department of Pathology) and 'Motor control in pyramidal and extrapyramidal disorders' (with the Departments of Physiology and Orthopaedic Surgery). We are keenly aware of the extraordinary advances in understanding the nervous system made possible by basic research and new technologies, and the immense implications for more effective therapy of nervous diseases. We also perceive that disorders of the nervous system will constitute an urgent and demanding problem for Hong Kong society in the coming decade. However, the present organization and resources in any single Department will not enable us to meet this challenge. It was against this background that a group of basic and clinical neuroscientists of this University deemed concerted research efforts essential and last year proposed the establishment of an Institute of Basic and Clinical Neurosciences. Should this proposal be accepted by the University, neurological research in Hong Kong will enter a new phase, with greater contribution to the international effort in prevention and treatment of diseases of the nervous system.

Major Publications

Cerebrovascular disease

1. Yu YL, Moseley IF, Pullicino P, McDonald WI: The Clinical picture of ectasia of intracranial arteries. *J Neurol Neurosurg Psychiatry* 1982; 45: 29–36.
2. Huang CY, Chan YW, Wang R: Senile dementia and hydrocephalus due to carotid dolichoectasia. *Clin Exp Neurol* 1982; 19: 171–176.
3. Huang CY: Cerebrovascular disease in Hong Kong. *Jpn Circulation J* 1982; 46: 605–608.
4. Huang CY, Broe GA: Isolated facial palsy. A new lacunar syndrome. *J Neurol Neurosurg Psychiatry* 1984; 47: 84–86.
5. Huang CY, Lui FS: Ataxic-hemiparesis, localization and clinical features. *Stroke* 1984; 15: 363–365.
6. Huang CY, Chan KH: Pontine ataxic hemiparesis, a lateral penetrator syndrome? *J Neurol Neurosurg Psychiatry* 1984; 47: 1046–1047.
7. Pun KK, Huang CY: Rotatory seizures associated with occipital lobe ischaemic infarction: a case report. *Asian Med J* 1984; 27: 400–408.
8. Pun KK, Wang RYC, Huang CY: Cardiac embolic cerebrovascular disease in Hong Kong 1979–1982. *Asian Med J* 1984; 27: 529–536.
9. Huang CY, Yu YL: Small cerebellar strokes may mimic labyrinthine lesions. *J Neurol Neurosurg Psychiatry* 1985; 48: 263–265.
10. Huang CY, Broe GA, Bruce C: Electronystagmogram is useful in the diagnosis of vertebrobasilar and carotid transient ischaemic attacks. *Ann Acad Med Singapore* 1985; 14: 44–48.
11. Huang CY, Yu YL, Woo E, Chan FL: Cerebral haemorrhage in a southern Chinese urban population. *Functional Neurol* 1986; 1: 213–221.
12. Huang CY, Woo E, Yu YL, Chan FL: When is sensorimotor stroke a lacunar syndrome? *J Neurol Neurosurg Psychiatry* 1987; 50: 720–726.
13. Tsoi M, Huang CY, Lee AOM, Yu YL: Amnesia following right thalamic haemorrhage. *Clin Exp Neurol* 1987; 23: 201–207.
14. Yu YL, Chiu EKW, Woo E, Chan FL, Lam WK, Huang CY, Lee PWH: Dystrophic intracranial calcification: CT evidence of 'cerebral steal' from arteriovenous malformation. *Neuroradiology* 1987; 29: 519–522.
15. Lau S, Chan FL, Yu YL, Huang CY, Woo E: Cortical blindness in toxaemia of pregnancy -findings on computed tomography. *Br J Radiology* 1987; 60: 347–349.
16. Woo E, Huang CY, Chan FL, Yu YL: Claude's syndrome: Clinical and CT correlations. *J Comput Tomogr* 1987; 11: 208–211.
17. Woo E, Huang CY, Chan V, Chan YW, Yu YL, Chan TK: Beta-thromboglobulin in cerebral infarction. *J Neurol Neurosurg Psychiatry* 1988; 51: 557–562.
18. Woo E, Chan YW, Yu YL, Huang CY: Admission glucose level in relation to mortality and morbidity outcome in 252 stroke patients. *Stroke* 1988; 19: 185–191.
19. Woo E, Ma JTC, Robinson JD, Yu YL: Hyperglycaemia is a stress response in acute stroke. *Stroke* 1988; 19: 1359–1364.
20. Huang CY: Ischaemic crebrovascular disease 1987. *Hong Kong Practitioner* 1988; 10: 3011–3013.
21. Woo E, Chan YW, Yu YL: What happens to the stroke patient? *Hong Kong Practitioner* 1988; 10: 3459–3471.

22. Huang CY, Woo E, Yu YL, Chan FL: Lacunar syndromes due to brainstem infarct and haemorrhage. *J Neurol Neurosug Psychiatry* 1988; 51: 509–515.

23. Yu YL, Yeung DWS, Woo E, Chiu EKW, Huang CY, Chan YW, Lau-Wong MMM: Subcortical arteriosclerotic encephalopathy: a clinical and radionuclide scintiscan study. *Acta Neurol Scand* 1988; 77: 486–492.

24. Lee AOM, Yu YL, Tsoi M, Woo E, Chang CM: Subcortical arteriosclerotic encephalopathy — A controlled psychometric study. *Clin Neurol Neurosurg* 1989; 91: 235–241.

25. Wong VCN, Yu YL, Liang R, Tso WK, Li A, Chan TK: Cerebral thrombosis in β-Thalassemia-Hemoglobin E disease. *Stroke* (in press).

Demyelination, aging and degenerative disorders

1. Huang CY: Peripheral neuropathy in the elderly, a clinical and electrophysiologic study. *J Am Geriatrics Soc* 1981; 29: 49–54.

2. Huang CY, Broe GA: Aging of the brain: Clinical neurology and neuroepidemiology. In: *New Approaches to Nerve and Muscle Disorders* (eds. Tomkins JK, Westerman RA), Excerpta Medica International Congress Series, 1981; 546: 254–261.

3. Huang CY, Mackenzie RA, Creasey H: Neurophysiological evidence of aging in Down's syndrome. *Clin Exp Neurol* 1982; 19: 139–146.

4. Chin D, Yu YL, Huang CY: The use of lisuride in severe Parkinson's disease. *Clin Exp Neurol* 1986; 22: 63 69.

5. Wong VCN, Yu YL, Chan-Lui WY, Woo E, Yeung CY: Ataxia telangiectasia in Chinese children — A clinical and electrophysiological study. *Clin Neurol Neurosurg* 1987; 89: 137–144.

6. Hawkins BR, Yu YL, Woo E, Huang CY: No apparent association between HLA and multiple sclerosis in Southern Chinese. *J Neurol Neurosurg Psychiatry* 1988; 51: 443–445.

7. Yu YL, Woo E, Hawkins BR, Ho HC, Huang CY: Multiple sclerosis amongst Chinese in Hong Kong. *Brain* (in press).

Drug effects

1. Yu YL, du Boulay GH: Is there an increased risk of early side effects of metrizamide in post-myelogram computed tomography? *Neuroradiology* 1984; 26: 399–403.

2. Yu YL, du Boulay GH, Paul E: Influence of certain factors on the manifestations of the adverse effects of metrizamide myelography. *Neuroradiology* 1986; 28: 339–343.

3. Pan HYM, Huang CY: Alternating skew deviation associated with Mandrax overdosage. *Aust NZ J Med* 1984; 14: 265–266.

4. Chan YW: Brainstem auditory and visual evoked responses in chronic alcoholics. M Med Thesis. University of Sydney, 1986.

5. Chan YW, McLeod JG, Tuck RR, Walsh JC, Feary PA: Visual evoked responses in chronic alcoholics. *J Neurol Neurosurg Psychiatry* 1986; 49: 845–850.

6. Chan YW, McLeod JG, Tuck RR, Feary PA: Brain stem auditory evoked responses in chronic alcoholics. *J Neurol Neurosurg Psychiatry* 1985; 48: 1107–1112.

7. Hammond SR, Yiannikas C, Chan YW: A comparison of brainstem auditory evoked responses evoked by rarefaction and condensation stimulation in control subjects and in patients with Wernicke-Korsakoff syndrome and multiple sclerosis. *J Neurol Sci* 1986; 74: 177–190.

8. Yu YL, Huang CY, Chin D, Woo E, Chang CM: Interaction between carbamazepine and dextropropoxyphene. *Postgrad Med J* 1986; 62: 231–233.

9. Chan YW, Woo E, Yu YL: Chronic effects of phenytoin on brainstem auditory evoked potentials in man. *Electroencephalogr Clin Neurophysiol* (in press).

Dysphasia in Chinese

1. Huang CY: Aphasia in Chinese. In: *Psychological Research in Chinese Language* (eds. Kao HSR, Chang CM), Wen Hoe Co Ltd., 1982; pp. 183–190.

2. Huang CY: Reading and writing disorders in Chinese — Some theoretical issues. In: *Psychological studies of the Chinese Language*

(eds. Kao HSR, Hoosain R), Chinese Language Society of Hong Kong, 1984, pp. 39–56.

3. Huang CY, Lau WK: Semantic locked-in dysphasia: relatively preserved reading and writing in a case of global dysphaisa. *J Neurolinguistics* 1985; 1: 193–208.

Epilepsy

1. Shorvon SD, Gilliatt RW, Cox TCS, Yu YL: Evidence of vascular disease from CT scanning in late onset epilepsy. *J Neurol Neurosurg Psychiatry* 1984; 47: 225–230.
2. Woo E, Chan YM, Yu YL, Chan YW, Huang CY: If a well-stabilized epileptic patient has a subtherapeutic anticonvulsant level, should the dose be increased? A randomised prospective study. *Epilepsia* 1988; 29: 129–139.

Infections

1. Chau PY, Huang CY, Kay R: Streptococcus suis meningitis: an important underdiagnosed disease in Hong Kong. *Med J Aust* 1983; 1: 414–417.
2. Chan KH, Chau PY, Wang RYC, Huang CY: Meningitis due to flavobacterium meningosepticum after transphenoidal hypophysectomy with recovery. *Surg Neurol* 1983; 20: 294–296.
3. Wang C, Huang CY, Chan PH, Preston P, Chau PY: Transerse myelitis associated with larva migrans: findings of larva in cerebrospinal fluid. *Lancet* 1983; 1: 423.
4. Chang CM, Chan FL, Yu YL, Huang CY, Woo E: Tuberculous meningitis associated with meningeal tuberculoma. *J Roy Soc Med* 1986; 79: 486–487.
5. Yu YL, Chow WH, Humphries MJ, Wong RWS, Gabriel M: Cryptic miliary tuberculosis. *Q J Med* 1986; 59: 421–428.
6. Chang CM, Woo E, Yu YL, Huang CY, Chin D: Herpes zoster and its neurological complications. *Postgrad Med J* 1987; 63: 85–89.
7. Chan YW, Ho HC, Kay CS, Li SW, Ip YM: Creutzfeldt-Jakob disease in Hong Kong – a case report. *J Neurol Sci* 1987; 80: 143–152.

8. Kwong YL, Yu YL, Chan FL, Lam KSL, Woo E, Huang CY: High-dose ketoconazole in cerebral aspergilloma. *Clin Neurol Neurosurg* 1987; 89: 193–196.
9. Leung R, Woo E, Yu YL, Huang CY: Listeria brain abscess associated with steroid therapy: successful non-surgical treatment. *Clin Exp Neurol* 1987; 24: 181–186.
10. Yu YL, Lau YN, Woo E, Wong KL, Tse B: Cryptococcal infection of the nervous system. *Q J Med* 1988; 66: 87–96.
11. Yu YL, Woo E, Chan FL, Chan TYK, Chan GCY: Cerebral infraction in cryptococcal meningitis. *Clin Exp Neurol* (in press).
12. Woo E, Yu YL, Huang CY: Cerebral infarct precipitated by praziquantel in neurocysticercosis — A cautionary note. *Trop Geogr Med* 1988; 40: 143–146.
13. Kwong YL, Woo E, Fong PC, Yung RWH, Yu YL: Mollaret's meningitis revisited: report of a case with a review of the literature. *Clin Neurol Neurosurg* 1988; 90: 163–167.
14. Woo E, Yu YL, Huang CY: Local tetanus revisited. Electrodiagnostic study in 2 patients. *J Electromyogr Clin Neurophysiol* 1988; 28: 117–122.
15. Yu YL, Lam WK: Cryptic miliary tuberculosis in the tropics (Invited review). *Semin Resp Med* (in press).

Neoplasms

1. Yu YL, Crockard AH, Smith JJ, Harries BJ: Extraspinal ependymoma at the cervicothoracic junction. *Surg Neurol* 1982; 17: 160–162.
2. Chin DKF, To LB, Blumberg PC, Burrow DD, Juttner CA: Central nervous system relapse after bone marrow transplantation for acute myeloid leukemia. *Cancer* 1983; 52: 2236–2239.
3. Woo E, Yu YL, Ng M, Huang CY, Todd D: Spinal cord compression in multiple myeloma — Who gets it? *Aust NZ J Med* 1986; 16: 671–675.
4. Woo E, Chan YF, Lam KSL, Lok ASF, Yu YL, Huang CY: Apoplectic intracerebral haemorrhage — An unusual complication of cerebral radiation necrosis. *Pathlogy* 1987; 19: 95–98.
5. Woo E, Lam KSL, Yu YL, Lee PWH, Huang

CY: Cerebral radionecrosis — Is surgery necessary? *J Neurol Neurosurg Psychiatry* 1987; 50: 1407–1414.

6. Woo E, Lam K, Yu YL, Ma J, Wang C, Yeung RTT: Temporal lobe and hypothalamic-pituitary dysfunction after radiotherapy for nasopharyngeal carcinoma. *J Neurol Neurosurg Psychiatry* 1988; 51: 1302–1307.

7. Liang RHS, Woo EKW, Yu YL, Todd D, Chan TK, Ho FCS, Tso SC, Shum JST: Central nervous system involvement by non-Hodgkin's lymphoma. *Europ J Cancer Clin Oncol* 1989; 25: 703–710.

8. Huang CY: Paraneoplastic CNS syndromes. In: *Malignant Disease in the Elderly* (eds. Caird FI, Brewin T), Butterworth (in press).

Neuromuscular diseases

1. Yu YL, Murray NMF: A comparison of concentric needle electromyography, quantitative EMG and single fibre EMG in the diagnosis of neuromuscular diseases. *Electroencephalogr Clin Neurophysiol* 1984; 58: 220–225.

2. Kung A, Ma JTC, Yu YL, Wang C, Woo E, Lam KSL, Huang CY, Yeung RTT: Myopathy in acute hypothyroidism. *Postgrad Med J* 1987; 63: 661–663.

3. Jones SJ, Yu YL, Rudge P, Kriss A, Gilois C, Hirani N, Nijhawan, Norman P, Will R: Central and peripheral SEP defects in neurologically symptomatic and asymptomatic subjects with low vitamin B12 levels. *J Neurol Sci* 1987; 82: 55–65.

4. Hawkins BR, Yu YL, Wong V, Woo E, Ip MSM, Dawkins RL: Possible evidence for a variant of myasthenia gravis based on HLA and acetylcholine receptor antibody in Chinese patients. *QJ Med* 1989; 70: 235–241.

5. Gin W, Hawkins BR, Zhang WJ, Wong V, Yu YL, Dawkins RL: MHC associated bewtween antistriational antibody-negative myasthenia gravis in the Chinese. *Adv Neuroimmunol* 1988; 504: 513–515.

6. Myasthenia Gravis Research Group (Chief investigator: YL Yu). The Hong Kong Myasthenia Gravis Data Bank. *J HK Med Assoc* (in press).

7. Chang CM, Yu YL, Wong M, Woo E, Huang CY: Type 1 familial amyloid polyneuropathy in a Chinese family. *Acta Neurol Scand* 1989; 79: 391–396.

Spinal cord disorders

1. Yu YL, Stevens JM, Kendall B, du Boulay GH: Cord shape and measurements in cervical spondylotic myelopathy and radiculopathy. *AJNR* 1983; 4: 839–842.

2. Yu YL: Management of cervical spondylotic myelopathy. *Lancet* 1984; 2: 171–172.

3. Yu YL: The use of computerised tomography in cervical spondylotic myelopathy and radiculopathy. M.D. Thesis. University of Hong Kong, January 1985.

4. Yu YL, Jones SJ: Somatosensory evoked potentials in cervical spondylosis: correlation of median, ulnar and posterior tibial nerve responses with clinical and radiological findings. *Brain* 1985; 108: 273–300.

5. Yu YL, du Boulay GH, Stevens JM, Kendall BE: Morphology and measurements of the cervical spinal cord in computer-assisted myelography. *Neuroradiology* 1985; 27: 399–402.

6. Yu YL, du Boulay GH, Stevens JM, Kendall BE: Computer-assisted myelography in cervical spondylotic myelopathy and radiculopathy: clinical correlations and pathogenetic mechanisms. *Brain* 1986; 109: 259–278.

7. Yu YL, du Boulay GH, Stevens JM, Kendall BE: Computed tomography in cervical spondylotic myelopathy and radiculopathy — Visualisation of structures, myelographic comparison, cord measurements and clinical utility. *Neuroradiology* 1986; 28: 221–236.

8. Yu YL, Chin D, Wen HL, Woo E: Spontaneous spinal epidural haematoma. *Clin Neurol Neurosurg* 1986; 88: 131–134.

9. Stevens JM, O'Driscoll DM, Yu YL, Kendall BE, Ananthapavan S: Some dynamic factors in compressive deformity of the cervical spinal cord. *Neuroradiology* 1987; 29: 136–142.

10. Yu YL, Moseley IF: Syringomyelia and cervical spondylosis: a clinicoradiological investigation. *Neuroradiology* 1987; 29: 143–151.

11. Yu YL, Woo E, Huang CY: Cervical spondylotic myelopathy and radiculopathy (In-

vited review). *Acta Neurol Scand* 1987; 75: 367–373.

12. Yu YL, Leong JCY, Fang D, Woo E, Huang CY, Lau HK: Cervical myelopathy from ossification of the posterior longitudinal ligament (OPLL) – a clinical, radiological and evoked potentials study in six Chinese patients. *Brain* 1988; 111: 769–782.

Miscellaneous

1. Pang SF, Huang CY, Ng MT, He ZC: Plasma concentrations of melatonin and N-acetylserotonin in different age groups of human males. *Acta Physiol Sinica* 1985; 37: 492–496.
2. Huang CY: Medicolegal aspects of brain death, the problem in intensive care units. *Medical Progress* 1987; 14: 7–8.
3. Yu YL: Editorial: Brain death and related issues. *J HK Med Assoc* 1987; 39: 137–138.
4. Chan YW, Woo EKW, Hammond SR, Yiannikas C, McLeod JG: The interaction between sex and click polarity in brain-stem auditory potentials evoked from control subjects of Oriental and Caucasian origin. *Electroencephalogr Clin Neurophysiol* 1988; 71: 77–80.
5. Huang CY: Regional Neurology. In: *Neurology in Clinical Practice* (eds. Bradley WG, Baroff RB, Fenchel GM, Marsden), Chap 81, Butterworth (in press).

Y.L. YU and C.M. CHANG

ACHIEVEMENTS IN RENAL MEDICINE

Establishment of the Renal Unit

A unit specializing in the care of patients with end stage renal failure was first formally established in Tung Wah Hospital in January 1980. Initially only haemodialysis service was provided. To cope with increasing patient load, continuous ambulatory peritoneal dialysis (CAPD) was introduced in March, 1983. In the same month, in collaboration with the Government and University Surgical Units, renal transplantation was started in Queen Mary Hospital. In August, 1983, a satellite dialysis centre was opened in Aberdeen. It initially provided haemodialysis service alone but in August, 1986, CAPD training was also started.

Up to September, 1989, our unit has trained a total of 411 patients for CAPD and is currently caring for 60 haemodialysis, 260 CAPD and 120 renal transplant patients. It is one of the busiest renal units in Hong Kong.

Contributions to Medical Literature

Glomerulonephrits

In collaboration with the Department of Pathology, a study of the pattern of primary glomerulonephritis in Hong Kong has shown that IgA glomerulonephritis and minimal change nephropathy are most common (1). The pathology of IgA glomerulonephritis has been studied in detail (2 4) and the morphological features which predict the clinical outcome has been described (5). A 3-year control trial of antiplatelet agents has failed to show a beneficial effect on disease progression (6). The distinction between minimal change nephropathy and other forms of nephropathy which present with nephrotic syndrome was facilitated by the establishment of a simple radial diffusion technique for measuring selectivity of proteinuria (7). A study on the serum immunoglobulin pattern and complement level has revealed that the IgE level may be helpful in predicting steriod responsiveness in patients suffering from nephrotic syndrome (8). A recent study of the role of a T cell derived lymphokine has failed to confirm an earlier claim

that it is a useful predictor of steroid responsiveness (9). We have assessed some of the newer modalities of treatment in minimal change nephropathy including the use of pulse intravenous methylprednisolone and cyclosporin A but the results were not encouraging (10, 11). A recent review of our experience on mesangiocapillary glomerulonephritis has shown that this form of primary glomerulonephritis has a bad prognosis (12).

Systemic lupus erythematosus (SLE) is the most common cause of secondary glomerulonephritis in our unit (13). Some less well documented manifestations of lupus nephritis including acute renal failure secondary to cresentic nephritis and tubulointerstitial involvement have been studied in detail (14–17). A study of serum beta-2-microglobulin in patients with SLE has shown that it may be of value in monitoring disease activity (18).

We were first in reporting the strong association of hepatitis B infection and membranous glomerulonephrtis in Hong Kong Chinese (19). In collaboration with the Hematology Unit, we have shown that urinary antithrombin III and fibrinogen degradation products were increased in patients with diabetic nephropathy with impaired renal function thus providing evidence that intraglomerular thrombosis may play a role in disease progression (20).

Dialysis

We have described in detail our experience of the first 100 patients on CAPD (21) including 17 diabetics (22) and 9 patients with SLE (23) and have shown that this is a safe and effective form of renal replacement therapy. Peritonitis remained the major obstacle to the long term use of CAPD and in Hong Kong, interestingly showed a seasonal variation (24). We were the first to report the intraperitoneal pharmacokinetics of ofloxacin given orally (25) and have successfully used oral ofloxacin in the treatment of bacterial peritonitis (26). Its effectiveness was comparable to that of conventional intraperitoneal antibiotics (27). We have also reported the largest reported series to date of pseudomonas

(29), tuberculous (29), and fungal peritonitis (30) and have made recommendations on their management. The high incidence of tuberculous peritonitis correlated with a similar high incidence of systemic, frequently extrapulmonary tuberculosis among our CAPD population (31). A prospective study of eosinophilic peritonitis in our patients has shown that this self-limiting, allergic form of peritonitis occurs frequently and needs to be distinguished from the infective forms (32).

We have studied the transperitoneal transfer of calcium and magnesium in patients on CAPD using commercially available dialysate solution and found that during a 8-hour exchange, magnesium balance is always negative and calcium balance is negative using high dialysate glucose exchange (33). A study of the lipid metabolism in CAPD patients has revealed hypertriglyceridemia, reduced HDL-cholesterol concentration and low hepatic and lipoprotein lipase activity (34). Treatment with gemfibrozil partly corrected these abnormalities (35).

In collaboration with the Endocrine and Clinical Biochemistry Unit, we have studied the mechanism of hypoglycaemia induced by propanolol in haemodialysis patients (36) and have shown that propanolol inhibits glycaemic response by a post-receptor post-cAMP blockade (37) and induces hypoglycaemia by limiting the availability of free fatty acids as well as inhibiting hepatic glucagon-stimulated glucose output and that metoprolol, a selective beta-1-antagonist, may have less effect on glucose metabolism than propanolol in haemodialysis patients (38, 39).

Renal transplantation

We have shown that C-reactive protein is useful in the diagnosis of allograft rejection (40). A comparative study of renal transplant patients receiving cyclosporin A and azathioprine has revealed that that the former group of patients have lower potassium excretion (41) while the the latter group have higher mean corpuscular volume (42). A study of the clinical course of hepatitis B positive patients who have received a renal transplant has revealed that a significant percentage developed hepatitis but there was no evidence of infection with the delta agent (43). Our unique experience of transplanting kidneys from hepatitis positive donors to negative recipients under the cover of hyperimmune gamma-globulin has shown that this practice may be safe and allows the use of kidneys from hepatitis B donors who would otherwise be rejected (44). A protein loading test was found not to be useful in predicting the renal reserve of donor following graft nephrectomy (45). A survey of urinary tract infection occurring after renal transplant has shown that it is an important cause of morbidity but does not affect long term graft function (46).

In other areas of nephrology

We have conducted a double blind control clinical trial on norfloxacin versus cotrimoxazole in the treatment of urinary infection and have found it to be more effective (47, 48). This is likely to reflect the high incidence of resistance of urinary pathogens to cotrimoxazole in our patients (49). An open trial of pefloxacin, a newer quinolone, has shown that it is also effective in the treatment of urinary infection but the incidence of side effects is higher (50). We have compared the effect of nadolol and propanolol on renal function in hypertensive patients with moderate renal insufficiency and have found that nadolol has less adverse effect on renal function than propanolol (51). A comparative study of cimetidine, ranitidine and antacids on renal function in individuals with peptic ulcer has shown that H_2-antagonists do not adversely affect renal function (52). A study in rats has shown that silymarin, a membrane protective agent, has a marked protective effect on gentamycin induced nephrotoxcity and suggested that this drug may be useful in humans at risk of developing aminoglycoside nephrotoxicity (53). A number of case reports have described unusual and interesting forms of renal diseases, complications of dialytic therapy and renal transplantation (54–65).

References

1.   Chan MK, Yin PD, Chan KW: Primary glomerulonephritis in Hong Kong. *Int J Urol Nephrol* 1988; 20(4): 413–420.
2.   NG WL, Chang CW, Yeung CK, Hua ASP: The pathology of primary IgA glomeru-

lonephritis — A renal biopsy study. *Pathology* 1981; 13: 137–143.

3. NG WL, Chang KW, Yeung CK, Kwan S: Peripheral glomerular capillary wall lesions in IgA nephropathy and their implications. *Pathology* 1984; 16(3): 324–332.

4. Cheng IKP, Chan KW, Chan MK: IgA nephropathy and steroid responsive nephrotic syndrome. The disappearance of mesangial IgA deposits following steroid induced remission. *Am J Kidney Dis* (in press).

5. Ng WL, Loke SL, Yeung CK, Kwan S, Chan KW, Chan MK: Clinical and histopathological predictors of progressive disease in IgA nephropathy. *Pathology* 1986; 18(1): 29–34.

6. Chan MK, Kwan SYL, Chan KW, Yeung CK: Controlled trial of anti platelet agents in mesangial IgA glomerulonephritis. *Am J Kidney Dis* 1987; 9: 417–421.

7. Jones BM, Hua ASP: A simple radial diffusion technique for measuring selectivity of proteinuria. *J Clin Path* 1980; 33(6): 598–599.

8. Chan MK, Chan KW, Jones BM: Immunoglobulins (IgG, IgA, IgM, IgE): and complement components (C3, C4) in nephrotic syndrome due to minimal change and other forms of glomerulonephritis, a clue for steroid therapy? *Nephron* 1987; 47: 125–130.

9. Cheng IKP, Jones BM, Chan PCK, Chan MK: The role of serum immune response suppressor lymphokine in the prediction of steroid responsiveness in idiopathic nephrotic syndrome. *Clin Nephrol* (in press).

10. Yeung CK, Wong KL, Ng WL: Intravenous methylprednisolone pulse therapy in minimal change nephrotic syndrome. *Aust NZ J Med* 1983; 13: 349–351.

11. Chan MK, Cheng IKP: Cyclosporin A in steroid-sensitive nephrotic syndrome with frequent relapses. *Postgrad Med J* 1987; 63: 757–759.

12. Chan MK, Chan KW, Chan PCK, Cheng IKP: Adult onset mesangiocapillary glomerulonephritis: a disease with a dismal prognosis. *Quart J Med* (New Series) (in press).

13. Chan WC, Ng WL, Lee AKY, Yu RYH: Lupus nephritis in Hong Kong. *Annals Acad Med Singapore* 1975; 4(2): 58–65.

14. Yeung CK, Ng WL, Wong WS, Wong KL, Chan MK: Acute deterioration in renal function in systemic lupus erythematosus. *Quart J Med* 1985; 56(219): 393–402.

15. Yeung CK, Wong KL, Wong WS, Ng MT, Chan KW, Ng WL: Crescentic lupus glomerulonephritis. *Clin Nephrol* 1984; 21(5): 251–258.

16. Ng WL, Chan MK, Wong KL, Wong RWS, Yeung CK: Unusual transformations of renal involvement in systemic lupus erythematosus. *Aust NZ J Med* 1985; 15: 69–71.

17. Yeung CK, Wong KL, Ng RP, Ng WL: Tubular dysfunction in systemic lupus erythematosus. *Nephron* 1984; 36(2): 84–88.

18. Yeung CK, Wong KL, Wong WS, Chan KH: β2-microglobulin and systemic lupus erythematosus. *J Rheumatol* 1986; 13(6): 1053–1058.

19. Sham MK, Pun KK, Yeung CK, Ng WL, Chang WK, Chan MK: Hepatitis B induced glomerulonephritis, fact or fiction. *Aus NZ J Med* 1985; 15: 356–358.

20. Chan V, Yeung CK, Chan TK: Antithrombin III and fibrinogen degradation product (fragment E) in diabetic nephropathy. *J Clin Path* 1982; 35(6): 661–666.

21. Chan MK, Lam SS, Chan PCK, Cheng IKP: Continuous ambulatory peritoneal dialysis (CAPD): Experience with the first 100 patients in a Hong Kong Centre. *Int J Artif Organs* 1987; 10: 77 82.

22. Chan MK, Lam SS, Chiu KW: Continuous ambulatory peritoneal dialysis (CAPD) treatment of diabetic patients in end-stage renal failure — Hong Kong experience. *J Diabetic Complications* 1987; 1: 11–15.

23. Chan PCK, Wong WS, Wong KL, Cheng IKP, Chan MK: Lupus nephritis patients on maintenance dialysis in Hong Kong. *Int J Artif Organ* (in press).

24. Chan MK, Chan CY, Cheng IKP: Climatic factors in the frequency of peritonitis. *Int J Artif Organs* (in press).

25. Chan MK, Chau PY, Chan WWN: Pharmacokinetics of ofloxacin in CAPD patients. *Clin Nephrol* 1987; 28(6): 277–280.

26. Chan MK, Chau PY, Chan WWN: Oral treatment of CAPD peritonitis with two dosage regimens of ofloxacin. *J Antimicrob Chemother* 1988; 22: 371–375.

27. Chan MK, Chau PY, Chan WWN: Oral treatment of CAPD patients. *Nephrol Dial*

Transplant 1988; 2: 194–197.

28. Chan MK, Cheng IKP, Chan CY, Ng WSF, Chan PCK: Pseudomonas peritonitis in CAPD patients. Characteristics and outcome of treatment. *Nephrol Dial Transplant* (in press).

29. Cheng IKP, Chan MK, Chan PCK: Tuberculous peritonitis complicating long term peritoneal dialysis — Report of 5 cases and review of the literature. *Am J Nephrol* 1989; 9: 155–161.

30. Cheng IKP, Fang GX, Chan MK, Chan TM, Chan PCK: Fungal peritonitis complicating peritoneal dialysis. Report of 27 cases and review of treatment. *Quart J Med* (New Series) 1989; 71(265): 407–416.

31. Chan PCK, Yeung CK, Chan MK: Tuberculosis in peritoneal dialysis patients. *Singapore Med J* 1988; 29: 103–104.

32. Chan MK, Chow L, Lam SS, Jones BM: Peritoneal eosinophilia in CAPD patients, a prospective study. *Am J Kidney Dis* 1988; 11(2): 180–183.

33. Kwong MBL, Lee JSK, Chan MK: Transperitoneal calcium and magnesium transfer during a 8-h dialysis. *Perit Dial Bull* 1987; 7: 85–89.

34. Chan MK, Yeung CK: Lipid metabolism in 31 Chinese patients on three 2-1 exchanges of CAPD. *Perit Dial Bull* 1986; 6: 12–16.

35. Chan MK, Pang WC, Leung JHB: Gemfibrozil improves abnormalities of lipid metabolism in CAPD patients: the role of postheparin lipases in the metabolism of HDL subtractions. *Metabolism* (in press).

36. Pun KK, Yeung KK, Young RTT: Propranolol-induced hypoglycemia in a hemodialysis patient. *Dial Transplant* 1986; 15: 195–196.

37. Pun KK, Yeung CK, Ho PWM, Lin HJ, Chan MK, Young RTT: Effects of propranolol and hemodialysis on the response of glucose, insulin, C-peptide and cyclic AMP to glucagon challenge. *Clin Nephrol* 1984; 21(4): 235–240.

38. Pun KK, Yeung CK, Young RTT: Effects of propranolol and metoprolol on glucose, cyclic AMP and insulin responses during pharmacologic hyperglucagonemia in hemodialysis patients. *Nephron* 1984; 39: 175–178.

39. Pun KK, Yeung CK, Chak W, Ho PWM, Chan MK, Lin HJ, Young RTT: Effects of selective and non-selective beta-blockers on the alanine and free fatty acids responses to glucagon challenge in haemodialysis patients. *Clin Nephrol* 1986; 26(5): 222–226.

40. Chan MK, Ye RG, Jones BM, Wong KK, Li MK: The use of C-reactive protein in the diagnosis of renal allograft rejection. *Singapore Med J* 1988; 29: 145–149.

41. Chan MK, Wong KK, Cheng IKP, Li MK: Clinical prevalence and significance of electrolyte disorders in cyclosporin A-treated patients. *Transplant Proc* 1988; 20 (Suppl 3): 705–708.

42. Fang GX, Chan PCK, Cheng IKP, Li MK, Chan MK: Hematological changes after renal transplantation. Differences between cyclosporin A and azothiaprine therapy. *Int J Urol Nephrol* (in press).

43. Chan MK, Chan PCK, Cheng IKP, Li MK, Chang WK: Hepatitis B infection and renal transplantation: The absence of anti-delta antibodies and possible beneficial effect of silymarin during acute episodes of hepatic dysfunction. *Nephrol Dial Transplant* 1989; 4: 297–301.

44. Chan MK, Chang WK: Renal transplantation from HBsAg positive donors to HBsAg negative recipients. *Brit Med J* 1988; 297: 522–523.

45. Chan MK: Protein loading test before and after kidney donation. *Aust NZ J Med* 1986; 16: 691–694.

46. Chan PCK, Cheng IKP, Wong KK, Li MK, Chan MK: Urinary tract infections in postrenal transplant patients. *Int J Urol Nephrol* (in press).

47. Chan MK, Wong WT, Yin PD, Cheng IKP: A double-blind controlled trial of cotrimoxazole versus norfloxacin in the treatment of urinary tract infection. *Br J Clin Pract* 1989; 43: 61–64.

48. Wong WT, Chan MK, Li MK, Wong WS, Yin PD, Cheng IKP: Treatment of urinary tract infections in Hong Kong: a comparative study of norfloxacin and cotrimoxazole. *Scand J Infect Dis* 1988; Suppl 56: 22–27.

49. Chan TM, Chan MK: Urinary tract infection in a female medical ward. *J Hong Kong Med Assoc* 1987; 39(4): 234–236.

50. Chan PCK, Wong WT, Cheng IKP, Chan MK: Clinical experience with pefloxacin in

patients with urinary treact infection. *Br J Clin Pract* (in press).

51. Pun KK, Yeung CK, Chan MK: Effects of nadolol and propranolol on renal function in hypertensive patients with moderately impaired renal function. *Br J Clin Pharm* 1985; 20: 40–44.

52. Yeung CK, Wong KL, Ng MMT, Lai CL: The effects of cimetidine, ranitidine and antacids on renal functions. *Clin Therapeut* 1984; 6: 620–624.

53. Chan MK, Ng WL: Silymarin ameliorates gentamycin nephrotoxicity. In: *Nephrotoxicity* (eds. Back and PH, Lock EA), Plenium Publishing Corp, 1989.

54. Chan WC, O'Mahoney MG, Yu DYC, Yu RYH: Renal failure during intermittent rifampicin therapy. *Tubercle* 1975; 56: 191–198.

55. Ng WL, Scollard DM, Hua ASP: Glomerulonephritis in leprosy. *Am J Clin Path* 1981; 76: 321–329.

56. Pun KK, Lui FS, Wong KL, Yeung CK: Retroperitoneal fibrosis associated with schistosoma japonicum infestation — An immunologically mediated disease? *Trop Geogr Med* 1984; 36(3): 281–283.

57. Chan DWS, Yeung CK, Chan MK: Acute renal failure after eating raw fish gall bladder. *Br Med J* 1985; 290: 897.

58. Yin PD, Chan KW, Chan MK: Minimal change nephropathy after acute decompression. *Br Med J* 1986; 292: 445–446.

59. Chan KW, Ho FCS, Chan MK: Adult Fanconi syndrome in K light chain myeloma. *Arch Path Lab Med* 1987; 111: 139–142.

60. Kwong YL, Chan KW, Chan MK: Acute post-streptococcal glomerulonephritis followed shortly by acute rheumatic fever. *Postgrad Med J* 1987; 63: 209–210.

61. Chan KW, Chan MK, Choy DTK: Nephrotic syndrome associated with angiofollicular lymph node hyperplasia. *Pathology* 1987; 19: 429 432.

62. Cheng IKP, Chan KW, Chan MK, Kung AWC, Ma JTC, Wang CCL: Glomerulonephropathy of Laurence-Moon-Biedl syndrome. *Postgrad Med J* 1988; 64: 621–625.

63. Chan PCK, To D, Chan KW, Cheng IKP, Chan MK: Cholesterol embolism causing acute renal failure after coronary bypass. *J Hong Kong Med Assoc* 1988; 40: 134–135.

64. Pun KK, Yeung CK, Chan TK: Acute intravascular hemolysis due to accidental formalin intoxication during hemodialysis. *Clin Nephrol* 1984; 21(3): 188–190.

65. Chan PCK, Chan KW, Cheng IKP, Chan MK: Living related transplantation in a patient with nail-patella syndrome. *Nephron* 1988; 50: 164–166.

Ignatius K.P. CHENG

ACHIEVEMENTS IN RESPIRATORY MEDICINE

Since 1974, the respiratory division has been served by the following physicians: Dr. Donald Y.C. Yu, Dr. S.Y. So, Dr. W.K. Lam, and Dr. Mary S.M. Ip. In addition, Dr. Jane C.K. Chan is completing her 2-year clinical training at Stanford, and Dr. George C.Y. Chan is now respiratory physician-trainee and will be furthering his training abroad next year. Over these years, the lung function laboratory has continuously evolved and modernized: e.g. from the water displacement spirometer (Godart Pulmotest) and Collins respirometer to the Gould 5000 IV Computerized Pulmonary Function Tests System (plus the Computerized Pulmonary Exercise Testing System), and from the dry bellows spirometer and the digital pneumotach and X-Y recorder to the portable electronic spirometer with real time test curve display. Improvement and expansion of our respiratory patient care during this period is also witnessed by the introduction of new diagnostic and therapeutic facilities (e.g. flexible fibreoptic bronchoscopy, histamine/methacholine bronchial challenge tests, allergy work-up, computerized volume ventilators with microprocessor controlled pneumatics and patient monitoring, computerized analysis of breathing patterns, nasal continuous positive airway pressure systems, oxygen concentrators for domiciliary oxygen therapy, pulse oximetry and end-tidal carbon dioxide monitoring, Nd-YAG laser therapy via fibreoptic bronchoscope, etc) and an increase of respiratory outpatient clinics from one per week before 1980 to 4 per week at present (general respiratory, asthma, respiratory oncology, and bronchiectasis).

Research has been an integral part of the work of the respiratory division in these 15 years. Epidemiological studies have established that bronchial asthma (1), bronchial carcinoma (2, 3), along with chronic bronchitis and emphysema and respiratory infections (including tuberculosis), are common respiratory problems in Hong Kong, whereas sarcoidosis (4) and asbestos-related diseases are relatively uncommon (5). The cumulative prevalence of asthma in adults was 0.5% (1), and research has been focussed on the effects of anti-asthmatic drugs to elucidate the pathogenesis of asthma, and the role of acupuncture. Sodium cromoglycate, a mast cell stabilizer, was found to be effective in asthma whether given by powder or by aerosol (6). The latter is preferred in Hong Kong where humidity is high, and the powder often clumps. The failure of inhaled verapamil and sublingual nifedipine to protect against allergen-induced asthma (7) would suggest that mechanisms other than the calcium ion flux-dependent mediator release (8) may be involved. Similarly, the ineffectiveness of ketanserin (a selective 5-hydroxytryptamine or serotonin blocking agent) on exercise-induced asthma suggested that serotonin had a limited role in its pathogenesis (9). More recently, airway inflammation with infiltration by inflammatory cells is thought to be central in the pathogenesis of asthma (10), and the effectiveness of inhaled corticosteroids has circumvented many of the problems associated with the chronic use of systemic corticosteroids (11). The demonstration of the efficacy of a twice daily inhalation regimen further simplified its use (12). A recent survey of asthma therapy in Hong Kong (13) has demonstrated a significant underuse of parenteral steroid in acute asthma and of topical steroid in maintenance therapy among general practitioners. This deficiency in management must be corrected as it may be a contributing factor for the rising asthma mortality in young males in Hong Kong in the past decade (14). By employing the techniques of histamine bronchial challenge and radionuclide gated lung scanning for examining the regional distribution of ventilation during bronchoconstriction, the pathogenesis of arterial desaturation in asthma was studied (15, 16). It was demonstrated that hypoxaemia seen in acute asthma was due to a shift of ventilation from base to apex and a reversal of normal ventilatory pattern. The role of acupuncture in asthma has been extensively studied (17, 18). An earlier study (19) showed that it did give bronchodilation though not as effective as isoprenaline inhalation. Acupuncture using trunk and forearm loci provided protection against exercise-induced asthma (20), whereas auricular acupuncture did not (21). Trunk acupuncture was also more effective than auricular acupuncture in reducing bronchomotor tone of stable asthmatics (17).

Bronchial carcinoma is the commonest lethal malignant disease in both sexes in Hong Kong, and accounted for more than a quarter of both male and female cancer deaths in recent years (2, 3). A prerequisite for any study of lung cancer is accurate pathologic and cytologic cell typing. In a study of 484 patients undergoing fibreoptic bronchoscopy between 1978–1982 (22), the cytologic cell typing accuracy was highest in squamous cell (SQ) and small cell (SC) carcinoma (87–92%), followed by adenocarcinoma (AD) (83%), and least accurate with large cell carcinoma (LA) (38%). The commonest cell type was SQ (39%) and AD (29%), followed by SC (12%) and LA (7%) (2). 90% of the male patients were chronic smokers (2, 23). Special features in our female patients included their high prevalence which ranked amongst the highest in the world, preponderance of adenocarcinoma (43%) and relative lack of association with smoking habit (about 50% of all cases and 60% of AD cases were non-smokers) (2, 3, 23). These observations have prompted studies to look into the possible aetiological factors. Passive smoking from a smoking husband was found to contribute to AD of the peripheral type (p=0.02) (3, 24). A recent collaborative study found that the risk ratio for passive smoking was 1.65 (p<0.01), with a significant dose relationship (25). The studies of other environmental inhaled agents (incense burning, kerosene stove cooking) (3, 24), tuberculous scars (26) and genetic factor such as HLA antigen frequencies (27) have all given negative results. On chemotherapy studies, good response rate was achieved mainly in SC carcinoma. Our first protocol was to use the MACC regimen (methotrexate/adriamycin/cyclophosphamide/CCNU) which produced 72% overall response rate and 11 months median survival in SC (cf. median survival of 1.5–3 months if untreated) (28). Unfortunately, 90% of responders would relapse within 3 years, and second-line salvage therapy by cisplatin + etoposide (VP16) gave a partial response rate of 40% only (29). Chemotherapy studies in non-small cell lung cancers have given disappointing results with the MACC (28), FuAM (Futraful/adriamycin/mitomycin-C) (30), FAM (5-fluorouracil) (31) and the escalated-dose FAM (Hi-FAM) regimens (32, 33). Hyper-

transfusion by red cell transfusion was found to result in less marked myelosuppression associated with chemotherapy (34), and warranted further study. Adjuvant immunotherapy by intrapleural BCG in operable non-small cell lung cancer patients did not improve survival at 5-year post-operatively (35), and gave significant complications of infections and chest pain instead (36). Our research in lung cancer has placed our respiratory division firmly in the international scene (37–44), and currently we are participating in a multicentre study of chemotherapy of SC lung cancer coordinated by the International Society of Chemotherapy.

An understanding of the pattern of bacterial isolates in lower respiratory tract infection and their antibiotic susceptibility is important for successful management of these patients. *S. pneumoniae* and *H. influenzae* are the commonest bacterial isolates from sputum in bronchopulmonary infections overall (45) and also in acute exacerbation of chronic bronchitis (46). Tetracycline was no longer the antibiotic of choice for treating these two organisms (58% and 23% resistance respectively) (46). Whereas only 3% of *H. influenzae* strains were β-lactamase producing (and thus ampicillin-resistant) in early 1980s (46), the figure has risen to 20% recently (47). In bronchiectasis, the commonest bacterial isolates from sputum were *Ps. aeruginosa, H.influenzae, H. parainfluenzae* & *K. pneumoniae* (47), so that amoxycillin appeared to be inferior to newer, broader-spectrum antimicrobials such as ofloxacin in treating these patients. And a collaborative study showed that the new antimicrobial imipenem-cilastatin gave a response rate of only 40% in febrile neutropenic patients with pneumonia as against an overall response rate of 70% (48). The first positive sputum culture for *Legionella pneumophila* was reported in 1983 (45), so was the first report of *Ps. pseudomellei* pneumonia (melioidosis) (49). It was subsequently shown that melioidosis could present as septicaemia particularly in elderly, diabetic or immunocompromised patients (50, 51), and that it was endemic in Hong Kong. About 14% of the subjects tested showed serological evidence of past infection (52).

Tuberculosis (TB) has remained an important health problem in Hong Kong. The first cautionary note on intermittent rifampicin therapy as a cause of renal failure appeared in 1975 (53). Unusual features of TB included the adult respiratory distress syndrome associated with miliary disease (54), bronchorrhoea associated with endobronchial disease (55), and local rib destruction simulating malignancy in pleuropulmonary TB (56). Endobronchial TB was of special interest, as half of the patients were afebrile, and chest radiograph was normal in 20% (57). As up to 85% of cases were sputum/smear negative for AFB, fibreoptic bronchoscopy became the investigation of choice, and often bronchoscopic findings were not unlike that of bronchial cancer. Apart from its use in endobronchial TB, fibreoptic bronchoscopy was also of great value in diagnosing sputum/smear negative pulmonary TB (58, 59) including immunocompromised patients with pulmonary infiltrates in whom pulmonary TB was found to be the second commonest cause after bacterial infections, and fibreoptic bronchoscopy carried a diagnostic sensitivity of 92% (60). Bronchial aspirate and lung biopsies were complementary (61), and bronchial aspirate culture, albeit taking a few weeks for the results, should be routinely performed in an area with high prevalence of TB such as Hong Kong, as it provided the exclusive diagnosis in 37 to 44% of all sputum negative cases undergoing bronchoscopy (61, 62). Serological diagnosis of TB has also been studied by assaying for IgG Ab to purified protein derivative by an ELISA technique (63). The initial findings showed that a positive result was obtained only when the disease was relatively long-standing or extensive. Also, it was not a reliable index of disease activity. Further studies are underway.

Colophony-induced asthma in electronic workers has been well described in the literature, but an unusual form of occupational asthma due to colophony was described locally in a vender removing feathers from poultry using a heated colophony-based mixture (64). The first report of asbestos-related diseases in Hong Kong — 3 patients with malignant pleural mesothelioma and 1 patient with asbestosis — also appeared in 1983 (5), and unusual extracellular birefringent laminated ovoid bodies were described in bronchial brushings and washings specimens in pulmonary talcosis (65). Bronchial provocation test was standardized for diagnosis of occupational asthma due to formaldehyde (66), which was shown to be most likely due to hypersensitivity with late asthmatic reactions following exposure. Still in the domain of occupational lung

diseases, acute exposure to dimethyl sulphate vapour was found to result in noncardiac pulmonary oedema with good functional recovery, but chronic bronchial hypersecretion continued (67).

Other respiratory clinical problems have also been addressed. Sleep apnoea, which is fairly common in the West, was first documented in our patients in 1985 (68). The use of systemic corticosteroid in chronic fixed airflow obstruction (CAO) is controversial. We showed in a double-blind cross-over controlled study that in patients with CAO, a course of oral prednisolone 40 mg daily for 2 weeks raised the forced expiratory volume in 1 second by $\geq$15% in 56% of the patients, and dyspnoea score and exercise performance also improved (69). However, no predictor of steroid responsiveness was identified. Another management controversy — suction drainage for pneumothorax — was also addressed, and it was shown that suction drainage up to 20 cm H_2O pressure did not have any advantage (70). In a study of myasthenia gravis, 5 respiratory problems were identified in 27 (46%) of 59 patients (71), namely abnormal lung function tests, respiratory tract infections, aspiration, acute respiratory failure requiring mechanical ventilation, and post-thymectomy pulmonary complications. Thymectomy was safe in second trimester of pregnancy (72). Interestingly, there was an increase (though non-significant) in prevalence of HLA B5 and B15 in adult myasthenic patients (73). Lung function tests have also been studied in various disorders: the forced expiratory volume in 1 second (FEV_1) and forced vital capacity (FVC), but not the total lung capacity (TLC) or transfer coefficient for carbon monoxide (KCO), were decreased in patients with β-thalassemia major receiving regular transfusion and desferoxamine (74); the VC progressively dropped while the TLC and KCO remained preserved in ankylosing spondylitis (75); the low lung volumes (FEV_1, VC, TLC) and high KCO in patients with mitral valvular disease were reversed after mitral valvular surgery because of decrease in cardiac size and reversal of pulmonary congestion (76); and the pre operative peak expiratory flow rates and PaO_2 values (along with age and serum albumin values) were identified as predictors for post-operative respiratory infection and respiratory failure in oesophago-gastric cancer surgery (77). Finally, exercise testing in thyrotoxicosis demonstrated gross hyperventilation (with respect to workload, oxygen consumption and CO_2 output) and hyperdynamic circulation, and that symptomatic improvement by β-adrenoceptor blockade was not associated with any real improvement of exercise performance till the hyperthyroid state was controlled (78).

In this era of molecular and cellular biology, it is natural that research in respiratory medicine should move in this direction. Earlier Epstein-Barr virus (EBV) studies in which we collaborated with the Department of Microbiology had shown that EBV DNA was detected by dot hybridization in washed exfoliative cells from bronchial lavages of 25(47%) of 53 patients undergoing fibreoptic bronchoscopy (79), and hence the lower respiratory tract appeared to be an important reservoir for EBV. Further co-culturing and fusion experiments demonstrated that the complete EBV was indeed present in exfoliative cells from the lower respiratory tract, which was latently infected with EBV (80). In bronchiectasis, mediators released from neutrophils may be important in the vicious cycle of inflammation, and non-steroidal anti-inflammatory drugs were shown to have no effect on the chemotactic response of mature neutrophils in vitro, but suppress chemotaxis progressively when given in vivo (81, 82). Further studies on the use of other anti-inflammatory drugs in modulating neutrophil chemotaxis and host response are in progress. The relevance of K-ras and other oncogenes in the development of lung cancer, particularly adenocarcinoma in our local population, is being studied. And when Dr. Jane C.K. Chan returns from Stanford, she will be fully equipped with the expertise to study cellular mechanism of acute lung injury.

Publications

1. So SY: Asthma — The Hong Kong perspective. In: *First East Asian Symposium On Asthma* (ed. Davies RJ), Excerpta Medica, Hong Kong, 1985; pp. 110–112.

2. Lam WK, So SY, Yu DYC: Clinical features of bronchogenic carcinoma in Hong Kong — A review of 480 patients. *Cancer* 1983; 52: 369–376.

3. Lam WK: A clinical and epidemiological study of carcinoma of lung in Hong Kong. M.D. Thesis, University of Hong Kong, 1985.

4. Lam WK, Nandi PL, Kung TM, So SY: Sarcoidosis in Hong Kong Chinese — A review of nine cases. *Asian Med J* 1983; 26: 712–715.

5. Lam WK, Kung TM, Ma PL, So SY, Mok CK: First report of asbestos-related diseases in Hong Kong. *Trop Geogr Med* 1983; 35: 225–229.

6. So SY, Yu DYC: Sodium cromoglycate delivered by pressurized aerosol in the treatment of asthma. *Clin Allergy* 1981; 11: 479–482.

7. So SY, Lam WK, Yu DYC: Effect of calcium antagonist on allergen-induced asthma. *Clin Allergy* 1982; 12: 595–600.

8. So SY, Ip M, Lam WK: Calcium channel blockers and asthma: A review. *Lung* 1986; 164: 1–16.

9. So SY, Lam WK, Kwan S: Selective 5-HT2 receptor blockade in exercise-induced asthma. *Clin Allergy* 1985; 15: 371–376.

10. So SY, Ip Mary SM, Kwan S, Lam WK: Changing concepts on pathogenesis of asthma. *Asian Pac J Allergy Immunol* 1985; 3: 217–220.

11. Ellul-Micallef R, Lam WK, Toogood JH (eds.): *Advances In The Use Of Inhaled Corticosteroids*, Excerpta Medica Asia Ltd., Hong Kong, 1987; 19 chapters, 210 pp.

12. So SY, Lam WK: Twice daily administration of beclomethasone diproprionate dry powder in the management of chronic asthma. *Asian Pac J Allergy Immunol* 1986; 4: 129–132.

13. So SY, Tse M, Ip M, Lam WK: Audit of asthma therapy in Hong Kong. *Proc 1st Congr Asia-Pac Soc Respir, Tokyo 1988*; p. 134.

14. So SY, Ng M, Ip M, Lam WK: Rising asthma mortality in young males in Hong Kong, 1976–85. *Proc 1st Congr Asia-Pac Soc Respir, Tokyo 1988*; p. 68.

15. Whyte K, Ip M, Kirby T, Muir AL, Flenley DC: Changes in arterial saturation and regional lung ventilation from histamine induced bronchoconstriction in chronic adult asthma. *Am Rev Respir Dis* 1987; 135: A311.

16. Ip M, Whyte K, Kirby T, Wathen C, Flenley

D: Arterial desaturation, hyperinflation and changes in regional lung ventilation during histamine bronchial challenge. *Clin Sci* 1987; 72 (Supp. 16): 85p.

17. So SY, Lam WK: Does acupuncture work in asthma? *Asian Pacific J Allergy Immunol* 1983; 1: 168–169.

18. So SY. Acupuncture in the management of asthma. In: *First East Asian Symposium On Asthma* (ed. Davies RJ), Excerpta Medica, Hong Kong, 1985; pp. 113–115.

19. Yu DYC, Lee SP: Effect of acupuncture on bronchial asthma. *Clin Sci Mol Med* 1976; 51: 503–509.

20. Fung KP, Chow OKW, So SY: Attenuation of exercise-induced asthma by acupuncture. *Lancet* 1986; ii: 1419–1422.

21. Chow OKW, So SY, Lam WK, Yu DYC, Yeung CY: Effect of acupuncture on exercise-induced asthma. *Lung* 1983; 161: 321–326.

22. Lam WK, So SY, Yu DYC, Hsu C: Fibreoptic bronchoscopy in the diagnosis of bronchial cancer: comparison of washings, brushings and biopsies in central and peripheral tumours. *Clin Oncol* 1983; 9: 35–42.

23. Lam WK, So SY: Cigarette smoking & histological types of lung cancer — A study of 843 Chinese patients in Hong Kong. *J H K Soc Community Med* 1984; 14: 9 15.

24. Lam WK, Kung TM, So SY, Bacon-Shone JH: Active & passive smoking, kerosene stove usage & home incense burning among female lung cancer patients — Case-control study. *Proc XV World Congr Dis Chest, Sydney 1985;* p. 33.

25. Lam TH, Kung TM, Wong CM, Lam WK, Kleevens JWL, Saw D, Hsu C, Seneviratne S, Lam SY, Lo KK, Chan WC. Smoking, passive smoking and histological types in lung cancer in Hong Kong Chinese women. *Br J Cancer* 1987; 56: 673–678.

26. Kung ITM, Lui IOL, Loke SL, Aung Khin M, Mok CK, Lam WK, So SY: Pulmonary scar cancer — A pathologic reappraisal. *Am J Surg Pathol* 1985; 9: 391–400.

27. Lam WK, Hawkins BR, Kung ITM, So SY. No association between HLA antigens and adenocarcinoma of lung in non-smoker female patients in Hong Kong. *Br J Dis Chest* 1986; 80: 370–374.

28. Lam WK, So SY, Ng RP, Yu DYC: Four-drug combination chemotherapy in inoperable bronchial cancer: methotrexate, adriamycin, cyclophosphamide and lomustine. *Proc 13TH Internat Congr Chemotherapy* (eds. Spitzy & Karrer), Egermann, Vienna, 1983; 248: 114–117.

29. Lam WK, Ip MSM, Chan JCK, So SY: Second-line chemotherapy of small cell lung cancer with cisplatin and etoposide. *Lung Cancer* 1988; 4: A111.

30. Lam WK, So SY, Yu DYC: Futraful, adriamycin and mitomycin-C in the treatment of inoperable adenocarcinoma of lung. In: *Proc 7TH Asia-Pac Congr Dis Chest* (eds. Nandi & Lam), Hong Kong, 1981; pp. 311–314.

31. Lam WK, So SY, Ip M, Yu DYC: Cyclic combination chemotherapy in advanced adenocarcinoma of the lung — Comparison of two FAM schedules. *Cancer Chemother Pharmacol* 1985; 14: 282–283.

32. Lam WK, So SY, Kung TM, Ip M: High-dose 5-fluorouracil, adriamycin and mitomycin-C chemotherapy for advanced adenocarcinoma of the lung. In: *Recent Advances in Chemotherapy* (ed. Ishigami J), Anticancer Section, University of Tokyo Press, Tokyo, 1985, pp. 1156–1157.

33. Lam WK, So SY, Kung TM, Sham MK, Ip M: 5-fluorouracil, adriamycin and mitomycin-C (FAM) chemotherapy in advanced adenocarcinoma of the lung: comparison of two dosage schedules. *Cancer Chemother Pharmacol* 1987; 19: 269–271.

34. Lam WK, So SY, Ng RP, Yu DYC: Can hypertransfusion attenuate myelosuppression associated with systemic chemotherapy in patients with inoperable lung cancer? — Report of a randomised controlled study. *Med Pediatr Oncol* 1983; 11: 343–346.

35. Law MR, Lam WK, Hodson ME: Post-operative intrapleural BCG in lung cancer. *Eur J Cancer Clin Oncol* 1988; 24: 1527–1528.

36. Law MR, Lam WK, Studdy PR, Pugsley WB, Hodson ME: Complications of intrapleural BCG in the treatment of operable non-small cell bronchial carcinoma. *Br J Dis Chest* 1982; 76: 151–156.

37. Lam WK: Bronchial carcinoma in Chinese women in Hong Kong. Chronicle, *Proc Roy Coll Physicians Edin* 1985; 15: 268–269.

38. Lam WK: Lung cancer international survey

— Hong Kong. *Lung Cancer* 1986; 2: 196–198.

39. Lam WK: The epidemiology of lung cancer in Hong Kong. *Asian Med J* 1987; 30: 347–352.

40. Lam WK: Chemotherapy of advanced carcinoma of lung in Hong Kong — A review of eight years. *Proc Guangzhou 2nd Symposium Lung Cancer Research*, Guangzhou Research Centre for Lung Cancer, 1987; pp. 98–101.

41. Lam WK: The experience of chemotherapy of lung cancer in Hong Kong. In: *Cancer in Asia And Pacific* (eds. Tjokronegoro A, Himawan S and Jusuf A), Yayasan Kanker, Jarkarta, Indonesia, 1988; 2 (Chapter 6): 665–671.

42. Lam WK, Du YX: Environmental inhaled agents and their relation to lung cancer. In: *Pathophysiology and Treatment of Inhalation Injuries* (ed. J Loke), Lung Biology in Health and Diseases Series (ed. Lenfant C), Marcel Dekker, New York, 1988; Chapter 10, pp. 423–451.

43. Kung ITM, Lam WK, Lam TH: Observer variability studies of the WHO classification of lung cancer. In: *Cancer Treatment and Reserarch: Lung Cancer* (ed. Hansen HH), Martinus Nijhoff Publishers, Boston, 1989; Chapter 4, pp. 53–69.

44. Lam WK, Ip MSM: Lung cancer: epidemiology and chemotherapy of advanced disease: the Hong Kong perspective (chapter). In: *Respiratory Malignancy* (ed. Bovornkitti S), Thai Publishers, Bangkok (in press).

45. Wong WT, Lam WK, So SY, Yu DYC: Clinical responses and bacteriological effects of intravenous and oral erythromycin in patients with bronchopulmonary infections. In: *Proc 13th Internat Congr Chemotherapy* (eds. Spitzy & Karrer), Egermann, Vienna, 1983; 107: 49–57.

46. Ling J, Chau PY, Leung YK, Ng WS, So SY: Antibiotic susceptibility of pneumococcus & H. influenzae isolated from patients with acute exacerbations of chronic bronchitis: prevalence of tetracycline-resistant strains in Hong Kong. *J Infection* 1983; 6: 33–37.

47. Lam WK, Chau PY, So SY, Leung YK, Chan JCK, Ip M, Sham MK: Ofloxacin compared with amoxycillin in treating infective exacerbations in bronchiectasis. *Br J Dis Chest* (in press).

48. Liang R, Yung R, Chau PY, Chan TK, Lam WK, So SY, Todd D: Imipenem/cilastatin as initial therapy for febrile neutropenic patients. *J Antimicrob Chemother* 1988; 22: 765–770.

49. So SY, Chau PY, Leung YK, Lam WK, Yu DYC: Successful treatment of melioidosis caused by a multiresistant strain in an immunosuppressed host with third generation cephalosporins. *Am Rev Respir Dis* 1983; 127: 650–654.

50. So SY, Chau PY, Leung YK, Lam WK: First report of septicaemic melioidosis in Hong Kong. *Trans R Soc Trop Med Hyg* 1984; 78: 456–459.

51. So SY: Melioidosis in Hong Kong. *Int Med* 1986; 2: 168–170.

52. So SY, Chau PY, Aquinas M, Gabriel M, Lam WK: Melioidosis — A serological survey in a tuberculosis sanatorium in Hong Kong. *Trans R Soc Trop Med Hyg* 1987; 81: 1017–1019.

53. Chan WC, Yu DYC, Yu RYH, Gabriel O'Mahoney M: Renal failure during intermittent rifampicin therapy. *Tubercle* 1975; 56: 191–198.

54. So SY, Yu DYC: The adult respiratory distress syndrome associated with miliary tuberculosis. *Tubercle* 1981; 62: 49–53.

55. So SY, Lam WK, Sham MK: Bronchorrhoea: a presenting feature of active endobronchial tuberculosis. *Chest* 1983; 84: 635–636.

56. Ip M, Chen NK, So SY, Chiu SW, Lam WK: Unusual rib destruction in pleuropulmonary tuberculosis. *Chest* 1989; 95: 242–244.

57. Ip MSM, So SY, Lam WK, Mok CK. Endobronchial tuberculosis revisited. *Chest* 1986; 89: 727–730.

58. Lam WK, So SY, Yu DYC: Fibreoptic bronchoscopy: analysis of results in 1450 Chinese patients in Hong Kong. *Chin Med J* 1983; 96: 737–742.

59. So SY, Lam WK, Yu DYC: Rapid diagnosis of suspected pulmonary tuberculosis by fibreoptic bronchoscopy. *Tubercle* 1982; 63: 195–200.

60. Chan JC, So SY, Lam WK, Ip M: High incidence of pulmonary tuberculosis in the non-HIV infected immunocompromized patients in Hong Kong. *Chest* (in press).

61. Lam WK, So SY, Chau PY, Yu DYC: Comparison of bronchial aspirate and transbron-

chial biopsy by fibreoptic bronchoscopy in the diagnosis of sputum smear-negative pulmonary tuberculosis. *Eur J Resp Dis* 1983; 64: 586.

62. Ip M, Chau PY, So SY, Lam WK: Value of routine bronchial aspirate culture at fibreoptic bronchoscopy for the diagnosis of M. tuberculosis infection. *Tubercle* (in press).

63. Chau PY, Wan KC, Ng WS, So SY, Lau WY, Fan ST, Lee DKY: Enzyme-linked immuno-sorbent assay (ELISA) of antibodies to purified protein derivative (PPD) in the diagnosis of active tuberculosis: Evaluation of its potential and limitation in a high prevalence area. *Trop Geogr Med* 1987; 39: 228–232.

64. So SY, Lam WK, Yu DYC: Colophony-induced asthma in a poultry vender. *Clin Allergy* 1981; 11: 395–399.

65. Kung TM, Johnson JB, So SY, Lam WK, Hsu C: Blue bodies in cytology specimens in a case of pulmonary talcosis. *Am J Clin Pathol* 1984; 81: 675–678.

66. Burge PS, Harries MG, Lam WK, O'Brian IM, Patchett PA: Occupational asthma due to formaldehyde. *Thorax* 1985; 40: 255–260.

67. Ip M, Wong KL, Wong KF, So SY: Lung injury in dimethyl sulphate poisoning. *J Occup Med* 1989; 31: 141–143.

68. Ip M, So SY, Lam WK: Obstructive sleep apnoea syndrome — A rare entity in Hong Kong Chinese? *J H K Med Ass* (in press).

69. Lam WK, So SY, Yu DYC: Response to oral corticosteroids in chronic airflow obstruction. *Br J Dis Chest* 1983; 77: 189–198.

70. So SY, Yu DYC: Catheter drainage of spontaneous pneumothorax: suction or no suction, early or late removal? *Thorax* 1982; 37: 46–48.

71. Ip MSM, So SY, Lam WK. Respiratory problems in myasthenia gravis. *Ann Acad Med* 1985; 14: 442–445.

72. Ip MSM, So SY, Lam WK, Tang LCH, Mok CK. Thymectomy in myasthenia gravis during pregnancy. *Postgrad Med J* 1986; 62: 473–474.

73. Hawkins BR, Ip M, Lam KSL, Ma JTC, Chan-Lui WY, Young RTT, Hawkins RL:

74. Fung KP, Chow OKW, So SY, Yuen PMB: Pulmonary function in thalassemia major. *J Pediatr* 1987; 111: 534–537.

75. Ip M, So SY, Lam WK, Ho E: The lungs in ankylosing spondylitis. *J West Pac Ortho Ass* 1988; 25: 25–28.

76. Lam WK, Wang RYC, Mok CK, So SY, Nandi PL, Lee WT: Mitral valvular replacement in patients with impaired respiratory reserve. In: *Proc VIII Asia-Pac Congr Dis Chest*, JCS Inc., Tokyo, 1983; p. 300.

77. Fan ST, Lau WY, Yip WC, Poon GP, Yeung O, Lam WK, Wong KK: Prediction of post-operative pulmonary complications in oesophago-gastric cancer surgery. *Br J Surg* 1987; 74: 408–410.

78. Yu DYC: On the physiological response to exercise in thyrotoxicosis: effect of β-adreno-ceptor blockade and antithyroid treatment. M.D. Thesis, University of Hong Kong, 1982.

79. Lung ML, Lam WK, So SY, Lam WP, Chan KH, Ng MH. Evidence that respiratory tract is major reservoir for Epstein-Barr virus. *Lancet* 1985; i: 889–892.

80. Almond J, Lung M, So SY, Lam WK, Ng MH: Epstein-Barr virus in the lower respiratory tract. In: *Epstein-Barr Virus And Human Diseases* (eds. Levine PH *et al*), The Humana Press, New Jersey, 1987; pp. 123–124.

81. Ip M, Lomas D, Shaw J, Burnett D, Stockley RA: The effect of non-steroidal anti-inflammatory agents on neutrophil chemotaxis. *Am Rev Respir Dis* 1989; 139: A304.

82. Ip M, Shaw J, Burnett D, Stockley RA: Effect of anti-inflammatory agents on neutrophil chemotactic response in vitro & in vivo. *Thorax* 1989; 44: 320.

W.K. LAM and Mary S.M. IP

EPILOGUE

It is always difficult to be the last speaker on an occasion such as this. Those who have spoken before have covered all the ground and there is little wisdom left to proclaim. T.K. Chan in his eloquent prologue, has given a comprehensive account of the outstanding achievements of David Todd, the man we honour today, during his long and fruitful career spanning over three and a half decades. The scientific seminar given by his colleagues this afternoon bears witness to the development and accomplishment of the department during his tenure as head from 1974–1989. The rebel that I am on this occasion too, I think I should once again abide by the law laid down by David Todd for the department 'The lady should have the last word'.

This task is not as impossible as I first imagined. For David Todd is no ordinary person, and in our long association as friends, fellow students and colleagues I have come to know him almost as well as myself. We first met in 1950 when I entered Queen Mary Hospital as the then 4th year medical student. It was a Thursday morning teaching clinic. David and I were called out by the late Professor McFadzean to stand in front of the class to discuss a patient who suffered from infective endocarditis. I was struck by the depth and breadth of his knowledge, his analytical and methodical approach and his precise and thoughtful answers. In fact he saved the day for me. Professor McFadzean was so pleased that he had at last found his perfect pupil — and successor to be — that he forgave me for all the silly mistakes I made that morning. The same characteristics evident as a young lad grew and blossomed as David graduated and advanced in his professional career. His exceptional industry, perseverance and searching mind are legendary. But this is not all. He brings to his teaching a sense of mission, to his clinical practice a living example of Hippocrates, to his research a happy marriage of astute clinical observation and scientific curiosity. He injects vision, honesty and fairness into his administrative duties as a leader or as a member of a team. These are rare qualities which, I am sure, have been responsible for his reputation as the best teacher in the department, a popular doctor, a distinguished researcher and a much sought after Committee member inside and outside the University.

It is a rare honour to be invited by the University Council to stay beyond the normal retirement age. We are pleased that David has accepted the invitation. These are difficult and challenging times for Hong Kong and more so for the universities and the medical profession. To compensate for the massive brain drain we have to increase student intake yet continue to improve the quality of undergraduate and postgraduate education. To improve the health care delivery and to accelerate the pace of self-reliance, we are taking steps to reorganize the management of hospitals and consolidate the structure of postgraduate professional training. In both ventures vital to the continuing prosperity and stability of Hong Kong, David will no doubt make a significant contribution through his participation in the University and Polytechnic Grants Committee, Provisional Hospital Authority's Working Party on Teaching Hospitals, Hong Kong College of Physicians and the future Academy of Medicine.

David is not actually retiring from the University today. He is only branching out to give more of his energy and wisdom to matters outside the Department of Medicine. When in due course he does retire, I am sure that he will be gratified with his achievements and what he has done for Hong Kong's education and medical profession, and that blessed with a good health and an optimistic personality, David will be able to enjoy life with happiness and satisfaction.

Rosie T.T. YOUNG